Contemporary Ethical Dilemmas in Assisted Reproduction

Contemporary Ethical Dilemmas in Assisted Reproduction

Edited by

Françoise Shenfield MA

Reproductive Medicine Unit
Elizabeth Garrett Anderson Obstetric Hospital
London, UK

Claude Sureau

Emeritus Professor of Obstetrics and Gynecology
Institute Theramex
Paris, France

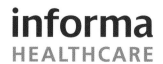

© 2006 Informa Healthcare, an imprint of Informa UK Limited

First published in the United Kingdom in 2006 by Informa Healthcare, an imprint of Informa UK Limited, 2 Park Square, Milton Park, Abingdon, Oxon OX14 4RN

Tel.: +44 (0)20 7017 6000
Fax: +44 (0)20 7017 6699
E-mail: info.medicine@tandf.co.uk
Website: http://www.tandf.co.uk/medicine

A CIP record for this book is available from the British Library.

Library of Congress Cataloging-in-Publication Data

Data available on application

ISBN10: 0-415-37131-7
ISBN13: 978-0-415-37131-5

Distributed in North and South America by

Taylor & Francis
6000 Broken Sound Parkway, NW, (Suite 300)
Boca Raton, FL 33487, USA

Within Continental USA
Tel.: 1(800)272-7737; Fax: 1(800)374-3401
Outside Continental USA
Tel.: (561)994-0555; Fax: (561)361-6018
E-mail: orders@crcpress.com

Distributed in the rest of the world by
Thomson Publishing Services
Cheriton House
North Way
Andover, Hampshire SP10 5BE, UK
Tel.: +44 (0)1264 332424
E-mail: tps.tandfsalesorder@thomson.com

Composition by Parthenon Publishing

Printed and bound by Antony Rowe Ltd., Chippenham, Wiltshire, UK

Contents

List of contributors

Charles Babinet
Unité de Biologie du Développement, Institut Pasteur, Paris, France

Gulam Bahadur
Department of Obstetrics and Gynaecology, Royal Free and UCL Hospitals, London, UK

Guido de Wert
Professor of Biomedical Ethics, Maastricht University, Research Institute GROW, Maastricht, The Netherlands

Joep P M Geraedts
Professor of Cell Biology and Genetics, Maastricht University, Research Institute GROW, Maastricht, The Netherlands

Carole Gilling-Smith
Consultant Gynaecologist, Assisted Conception Unit, Chelsea and Westminster Hospital, London, and Medical Director, The Agora Gynaecology and Fertility Centre, Sussex, UK

Gillian M Lockwood
Medical Director, Midland Fertility Services, Aldridge, UK

Guido Pennings
Professor of Ethics and Bioethics, Department of Philosophy and Moral Science, Ghent University, Ghent, Belgium

Gamal I Serour
Professor of Obstetrics and Gynecology, Al-Azhar University, Cairo, Egypt; Chairman, ERC of the Royal College; Chairman, FIGO Committee for Ethical Aspects of Human Reproduction and Women's Health; Secretary General of IFFS

Françoise Shenfield
Reproductive Medicine Unit, Elizabeth Garrett Anderson Obstetric Hospital and UCL Hospitals, London, UK; member of ESHRE Ethics and Law Taskforce; member of FIGO's Ethics Committee

Claude Sureau
Emeritus Professor of Obstetrics and Gynecology, and President, Institute Theramex, Bioethics, Women's Health and Society, Paris, France; former President of FIGO's Ethics Committee; member of the French National Ethics Committee

Gérard Teboul
Director du Centre d'Observation et de Recherche sur la Responsabilité et l'Autorité (CORRA), Université de Paris XII, and Law Professor, Université de Paris VII, Paris, France

Preface

This is the fifth time that we have had the pleasure of co-editing a book on the many dilemmas which we face in our profession.

Ten years after the first book, what has changed? Sometimes we feel that we have been full cycle and back again, with 'the great embryo debate' for instance. Sometimes we marvel that a new question has not been forecast in all these years of reflection.

So, what is new? One day there is (practically) a free-for-all in the practice of assisted reproductive technologies (ART), the next there is strict prohibition, as in Italy (a just or unjust comeuppance for the fantastic endeavors of a few?); some small progress (or is it 'plus cela change et plus c'est la même chose') with the recent legislation in France, where embryo research is still forbidden unless allowed in 'exceptional circumstances'; an important advance in the increased national and international debate about the ills of multiple pregnancies, with actual measures undertaken by professional or legislative or funding bodies (as in Belgium) in order to put a stop to the epidemic which we have created.

There are some matters which, sadly, are still present and which we wish would no longer need discussion, such as female genital cutting, or the discrimination (regarding both treatment and reproductive help) imposed upon HIV sufferers; yet other matters we may be bored with (yes, even us, the 'ethico-enthusiasts'), such as cloning. Is reproductive cloning 'a crime against humanity'? No, we feel that such language should be reserved for the many dramas and catastrophes seen in the 20th century and sadly still in the 21st, and outside the scope of this book, matters political and of human rights, without forgetting that the human right most disrespected to this day is that of every child to an education.

What is 'old' in this book is the notion of responsibility, which we hold dear in our respective professions, and personally. It is incorporated in the modern world in the context of human rights, of course, but also in the good old-fashioned way of what constitutes our duty (of care, or from one agent to another). What is new and satisfying? This includes the decrease in the incidence of multiple pregnancies due to ART in many countries; the ever-increasing responsible attitude of much of the media, who almost boycotted in 2003 a conference organized by a scientist claiming that the first cloned (as per the Dolly method) human embryo/fetus to be born was soon expected; the broad-minded attitude of official bodies such as the Human Fertilisation and Embryology Authority (HFEA), who admitted that they 'got it wrong' the first time around in the HLA tissue typing and preimplantation genetic diagnosis (PGD) debate and recently allowed the creation of 'savior siblings' in the UK, even if there is no genetic disorder to exclude in the future child, and who have confirmed the saying that 'only fools do not change their mind'; the enlarged Europe, which improves communication (as seen in the European IVF Monitoring Program/European Society of Human Reproduction and Embryology (ESHRE) figures of 2004 presented in Berlin) and therefore promotes better information for carers and recipients, and hence better care; the increased rate of literacy in many developing countries, which will again increase everyone's autonomy by better access to information.

These debates have informed our choice of chapters, and as ever we are grateful to the several colleagues and friends who have given their contributions to another book on the concerns that many of us in the field face, both at the clinical and at the research level.

Françoise Shenfield
Claude Sureau

Foreword

MORAL PHILOSOPHERS AGAIN EXAMINE THE ETHICS OF ASSISTED HUMAN CONCEPTION

They have done it again – Françoise Shenfield and Claude Sureau have organized another excellent book on the moral philosophy of assisted conception. Many of us, but not all, accept that the opinions of moral philosophers and of ethicists (if they are not one and the same) are of immense significance to our field of study. Perhaps more than most other topics, the establishment of human embryos *in vitro*, their care, their genetics, their birth and their situation after birth create a circumstance where morals and ethics reach a peak of intensity, especially since embryos can be transferred to other women, gestated in surrogate mothers and exposed to preimplantation genetic diagnosis and prenatal testing. Attendant embryologists, endocrinologists, geneticists and their clinical counterparts are now spread worldwide, so they all share similar duties to their patients. Many of them are deeply aware of their lack of any training in ethics, let alone moral philosophy. In these circumstances, we must respect how moralists are taught to think and form judgments on the most complex of issues. This book offers an example where two experienced thinkers have offered their latest observations on the scientific and clinical developments of assisted human conception. It is well worth reading.

In their wisdom, Françoise and Claude requested eight discussions, including their own, divided into three sections: The embryo – an entity worthy of respect; The intended parents and family welfare; and lastly The offspring and society at large. The opening chapter from Gillian Lockwood moves straight into the fray as it contrasts Kahlil Gibran's belief that 'Your children are not your children . . .' with the attitude of UK law implying that full-term fetuses do not exist and only at birth are they recognized as a single entity. In Western societies, a 'competent' mother can refuse to undergo life-saving medical or surgical interventions to save a baby. How about the early embryo? The UK Human Fertilisation and Embryology (HFE) Act conferred a special status on them at fertilization and held that they were neither objects nor possessions. Examples of cases in the High Court in London of contested ownership reveal the intensity of this complex situation, now under the care of the European Court of Human Rights. Other examples abound in a country as small as the UK, yet today the largest countries have entered the fray, so that numbers of complex cases will increase 50- or 100-fold. Many of these examples may concern law in combination with moral philosophy, and the mind boggles at the potential legal issues likely to emerge as we contemplate frozen-stored embryos, embryologists' mistakes, gamete donation and surrogacy, cloning, gene therapy and cell substitution.

Shenfield, Babinet and Teboul turn to modern developments, and especially to cloning. They stress the technical developments that had been thought to lead to successful human cloning in Korea and the formation of numerous stem-cell lines. Their article was written before the illicit facets of this Korean cloning were publicized. Clearly fascinated by the legal aspects of their study, they stress that it is the outcome of cloned children that raises peturbations and not the techniques themselves. To the scientist, the perspective is different, since one technique leads to another as with many new advances in this field. These authors are somewhat in error when they claim that cloning first captured public imagination quite recently, when in fact doom-laden authors debated the same topics 30 years ago, or that embryo stem cells were first isolated 20 years ago, when it was actually 50 years ago. They distinguish between President Chirac calling cloning 'a crime against the person' and the wider 'crime against humanity'. Cloning could raise issues on the meaning of 'human being' and 'human person', since the former may refer to a person who is being created and the latter to those already born. Asking the question: 'Where are we now?', they define the facts of cloning, stem cells, nuclear transfer, dedifferentiation, pluripotency and the other terms in widespread use today, a formidable list of ethical issues urgently needing philosophical and legal attention. Concentrating on legal aspects, they stress how jurists calling for cloning to be prohibited are passing rules before the science is done, which is the opposite way around to most ethical decisions on assisted reproductive technologies (ART). They describe the complex situation arising when France and Germany approached the UN about an international ban on reproductive cloning. With respect to ethics, these authors analyze the concept of a cloned child being judged in society as 'somewhat predetermined'. In contrast, stem cells have not invited such opprobrium, and a statement from the Australian State of Victoria that 'ES cells . . . are not the equivalent of an intact embryo . . .' has attracted their attention.

The third author, Gulam Bahadur, raises even further moral incongruities such as being a parent after one's death. Technically, this is an easy matter with present-day techniques in assisted human conception. The concepts under study are frozen-stored spermatozoa, oocytes and embryos. One very public case concerned a widow wishing to use the spermatozoa of her dead husband to conceive another child. The consequences for her were dire as she traveled through lawyers and judges in the UK and Europe, since the clear intent of the law is that the posthumous person must have given consent before he died, and this fact must be proven, yet the posthumous need to grant permission in this way is seldom if ever discussed among couples before they die. British law has achieved an added dimension with the declaration that private bodies should not interfere with privacy or family life unless to protect public health or morals. The latter is no easy task in mixed societies. Numerous cases have arisen, some being described in this chapter, and a notorious case in Australia concerned two living embryos whose parents died in a plane crash. The author describes many such heart-rending events occurring in his clinic, and comments on the potential harmful effects on children of bringing them into a home where one parent has died. These and many other examples witness the significance of the UK HFE Act in restricting the interference of public bodies in family life. Imagine the possible future effects of preparing gametes from stem cells!

The fourth author, Guido Pennings, debates the consequences of international parenthood via procreative tourism. He debates changes in the meaning of 'tourism', since people traveling afar for a child are certainly not tourists in the accepted manner, and prefers the term 'cross-border reproductive care'. This topic has been raised by the European Commission in its encouragement of people to travel to adjacent countries for medical care lacking in their own. The Commission is apparently not dealing with reproductive care, and the author speculates on this potential application. Semen samples may be delivered to a patient's home in a distant country, together with an insemination kit, and some US clinics have a branch abroad where they collect eggs, use the husband's spermatozoa for fertilization and then send the frozen embryos home for transfer. Reasons for such activities include a lack of availability of the necessary care in the home country or its very high costs. Too strict a law at home is another cause. In today's world, this kind of activity may become widely practiced, especially in Italy, in response to its passing a regressive law on infertility care. Risky treatments may be another compelling factor, or a refusal to treat social groups barred from care at home, e.g. lesbians or homosexuals. Obviously, richer people are at an advantage in gaining these treatments, which has long raised issues as to their 'loyalty' to their home country. Traveling abroad for treatment might have major consequences, such as for a couple returning home with a cloned child or two. The author also debates the international harmonization of legislation so that activities abroad may be resolved under the law of the home country. Seemingly, in Germany, researchers who travel abroad for research illegal at home can be tried in court when they return. Such cross-border reproductive care could entail major risks, e.g. raising costs of care in the foreign country, ignoring patients' rights, limiting informed consent and causing errors due to linguistic differences and to low (even unacceptable) standards of care. In Europe, two legal principles, namely freedom of movement of both goods and services, may confer a right for reproductive tourism. Thoughts such as these lead inevitably to the consideration that governments should not repress the rights of citizens to widely variable forms of health care, and whether flouting home laws by reproductive tourism does represent civil disobedience.

The fifth author, Carole Gilling-Smith, discusses risking parenthood in relation to HIV and hepatitis by using new reproductive technologies. Reproductive specialists must apply the four principles of medical ethics: do no harm, do good and respect autonomy and justice. Knowledge of a risk of familial illnesses, a satisfactory home environment and a multidisciplinary team are essential. These two illnesses differ in their impact on the risk to non-infected partners via horizontal transmission. Sperm washing or donor insemination have been recommended in the UK to avoid transmission from the man to his partner, and a European study identified no seroconversions in almost 5000 non-infected partners or children. Even so, a recent European task force recommended restricting assisted conception to serodiscordant couples. Many other issues emerge, including risks to other patients under care, infecting the scientific staff in a clinic and the risks of ovum donation in HIV-positive patients.

Françoise Shenfield and Claude Sureau contribute the sixth article regarding who is responsible for the welfare of the child. Commenting that this is usually left to the parents, they draw attention to the changes brought about by assisted conception and its stress on the welfare of the future child. Excellent clinical care has become paramount, avoiding the passage of a familial illness may become essential and certain couples may be prevented from conceiving (e.g. lesbians and homosexuals, but also those with serious familial defects). Methods such as forced sterilization for imbeciles were previously common and may still persist here and there, yet they have long disappeared from many countries. Legal UK terms include 'welfare' of the unborn child and 'best interests' of a born child. Risk is often difficult to judge, and medical doctors must maintain an open mind when assessing parental autonomy. Cases in which a highly damaged fetus was born rather than being aborted have involved judgments whereby the fact of its existence is a major benefit, which can affect attitudes in some legal cases. Psychosocial factors are equally complex, such as what happens to cryopreserved embryos when the husband dies, the right of a child to know his parents or the complexities that arise if a commissioning mother refuses to accept the baby from its surrogate mother. These and other examples have been associated with ART since its inception, and from even earlier times in relation to adoption. Such risks have led to debates as to whether assisted conception should be refused if the child's welfare is thought to be threatened. Various thresholds of damage and their acceptance have been postulated, and have led to conflicting interpretations of child welfare or the beliefs of a practitioner, among other factors. The UK HFE Act states that there should be a presumption of treatment unless evidence exists of serious mental, physical or psychological harm to a child or a sibling. Whether the clinician in charge can make such decisions is a matter of conjecture.

The seventh chapter, written by Guido de Wert and Joep Geraedts, discusses the ethics of preimplantation genetic diagnosis (PGD) for cases where hereditary disorders are not inherited according to a Mendelian pattern. These cases are sometimes called complex disorders. They arise from polygenic inheritance or combinations of genes and environmental factors. Long-term opposition has suggested banning PGD in cases where mutifactorial disorders or 'susceptibility' genes exist in the family. Grounds for refusal seem to be that environmental factors can be controlled, and that the disorders do not manifest until late in life. Concern for the children's self-image is also considered as a preventive factor. Philosophers such as Carson Strong stress that the physician's role is to help couples have a healthy baby, while Steinbock has argued for the force of reproductive freedom, e.g. a woman can abort a child even if it seems to others to be frivolous or trivial. A Canadian committee is scorned as being very weak in that their reasons for objection are incorrect, e.g. they proposed it is impossible that reproductive tests could provide 100% certainty, relevant environmental factors are unknown, all multifactorial disorders are late-onset, potential harm to the self-image of the children can be averted and varying gene penetrance can be accepted in many cases. The authors also criticize some limits of the arguments of Strong and Steinbock, and suggest that while a solution is exceedingly difficult to find, a number of relevant variables should be considered. These include the severity of the disorder, its age of onset and the degree of gene penetrance, so the strongest case for treatment is when the handicap is severe, therapy is impossible, it is early-onset and the gene disorder has complete penetrance. Allocating scarce resources to such irregular forms of expression is also a drawback. They suggest that three other aspects are significant, namely whether primary prevention is possible, whether residual genetic risks could persist after PGD and assessing the different intentions of couples who attend for genetic risk only as compared with those who attend for *in vitro* fertilization (IVF) alone. After describing typical cases under the various categories, the authors conclude that susceptibilities cannot be simply dismissed on ethical grounds, morally relevant variables should be considered and adequate counseling is essential.

The final chapter, by Gamal Serour, debates religious perspectives of ethical issues in ART. He contrasts the changes in this field of ethics to a more secular position in Western countries, but this is seemingly unnecessary in the Middle East where contemplation and mystery are essential. The role of reproduction in Western society, and perhaps most if not all others, varies widely, but is generally pro-child and pro-family formation. The author stresses the vast change wrought by the birth of the first IVF baby and the opening of human conception to scientific medicine. Each belief is assessed in detail, including Judaism, Christianity, Islam, Confucian–Taoist, Buddhist and Hindu. So much detail is provided that it is impossible to review all the complex reproductive situations in a Foreword!

Reading this book convinces me yet again that the complex issues of ART must be discussed and re-discussed until a measure of clarity is gained. Many of the older issues are largely solved, at least in law, although new advances in the offing will raise even wider issues about parentage, enhancing children genetically and extracorporeal pregnancy, to name but three. These new items are covered by each set of authors in the book as they discuss fundamental points of ethics and moral law. They have striven to clarify where we stand today, and perhaps where we may stand tomorrow. One point fills me with doubts, namely the necessity for a universal law to cover cloning and other complex problems. One glance at Europe's current strife regarding the ethics of ART should be sufficient to discourage any attempt at unity. Perhaps my response to the astonishingly diverse aspects of IVF described by the authors of this book stresses my own need for a greater understanding of and sympathy with this vast field of human endeavor. In the mean time, Françoise and Claude have again produced a book demanding careful reading and a disposition to understanding the problems of human couples facing so many diverse suggestions for their care. I send my deepest thanks to them.

R G Edwards

PART I

THE EMBRYO:
AN ENTITY WORTHY OF RESPECT

Chapter 1

Whose embryos
are they anyway?

Gillian M Lockwood

Your children are not your children.
They are the sons and daughters of Life's longing for itself.
They come through you but not from you,
And though they are with you, yet they belong not to you.

The Prophet by Kahlil Gibran

How different this is from the approach of the Ancient Greeks, who took the view that children (and one remained a minor in those days until the age of 30!) were the property of their fathers, who therefore exercised a right of life and death over them in early childhood and certainly during the neonatal period (the habit of exposing 'surplus' baby girls on the hillside as a form of infanticide is well documented).

UK law demonstrates a remarkable dissonance between the rights it ascribes to fetuses and the rights it ascribes to embryos. Even the full-term fetus does not 'exist' in UK law in the sense that until a baby is born it is not recognized as a separate entity from its mother. Its life may be terminated up to 24 weeks' gestation if healthy, and beyond that for compelling maternal reasons or if there is significant risk of handicap. As long as the mother-to-be is deemed 'competent' she has the right to refuse any or all medical or surgical interventions that could save the baby's life, even if her beliefs or fears seem irrational to those caring for her[1].

Under the terms of the Human Fertilisation and Embryology (HFE) Act (1990)[2], special status is accorded to human embryos from the moment of fertilization as befits their potential as possible people. Whether transferred or frozen, donated or experimented on, strict rules determine the conditions in which they are maintained, stored or ultimately disposed of. The Act makes it clear that embryos (like the gametes from which they are created) should not be treated as objects or possessions to which the normal rules of transactional commerce apply. Individuals may be 'compensated' for the trouble inherent in being gamete donors (in the UK currently £15 plus travel expenses per donation for sperm and egg donors). 'Egg sharers' may have all or most of the cost of their *in vitro* fertilization (IVF) cycle discounted in return for half or even more of their eggs, and the egg recipient is not 'buying' the donated eggs but rather paying for the medical and scientific skills necessary to provide the treatment. Couples or individuals who donate their surplus embryos are, at most, indemnified against the costs of storage, and a woman who receives donated embryos in a system akin to 'preimplantation adoption' is not purchasing the embryos any more than are adoptive parents buying the child they have placed with them.

So if embryos cannot be owned in the sense of being able to be bought and sold or even bequeathed in a will (!), why have the courts of law in the UK and elsewhere been quite so exercised about their disposition? The issue arises in the UK because the HFE Act stipulates that the informed consent of both parties who contributed gametes towards the formation of embryos must be ongoing for the embryos to be cryopreserved, continue in storage or be transferred up to the point of use.

Two cases of contested 'embryo ownership' (*NE* vs. *HJ* and *LH* vs. *WH*) came before the High Court in London in 2003, and one (*NE* vs. *HJ*) went to the Appeal Court and to the House of Lords, and is currently awaiting judgment from the European Court of Human Rights. In this chapter I intend to outline the two cases and draw parallels with similar cases heard in the USA and elsewhere. I endeavor to disentangle the complex web of issues relating to genetic identity, 'family' and rights which have resulted in contradictory and even counterproductive legislation being passed in the area of adoption and gamete donation. I hope to suggest a mechanism by which such cases may be resolved or, better still, avoided in the future and, perhaps more significantly, reduce the desperate waste and sorrow that result from over 90% of cryopreserved embryos being eventually discarded.

An unmarried couple, NE and HJ underwent fertility investigations after 18 months of primary infertility. These revealed that NE had early ovarian cancer, and the couple were advised that IVF with embryo cryopreservation was the only prospect for NE potentially achieving genetic motherhood, as a bilateral oophorectomy would need to be performed. At the time, NE was advised that egg cryopreservation was not possible. Six embryos were created and stored and NE underwent surgery, but the couple separated before any of the embryos could be transferred. HJ wrote to the fertility unit requesting that the embryos be taken out of storage and perished, as he was exercising his right under the Act to withdraw consent to their continued storage or use.

LH and WH were a married couple with two embryos in storage following an unsuccessful 'fresh' transfer as part of an IVF treatment cycle. The couple divorced before the frozen transfer was planned, and WH requested that the embryos be perished. LH, who was aged 37 at the time of the divorce, is subfertile due to polycystic ovary syndrome (PCOS), and wanted to have the frozen embryos transferred. LH has a 17-year-old daughter from a previous relationship.

In both cases the man now has a child from his new relationship, and both claim that it is not an issue of possible financial liability for a child or children born from their stored embryos, but rather that they do not wish there to exist children born to their ex-partners who would stand in the same genetic relationship to themselves as their own newborn babies.

Although the legal criteria of 'ownership' would not ordinarily be influenced by the personal circumstances of the claimants, there are significant differences between the two cases that may explain why strict application of the Act (which is quite unequivocal on the point of the need for continued joint consent for storage and/or use of embryos) proved so contentious. After all, in the case of Diane Blood and the use of sperm taken from her moribund husband, the Act was equally unequivocal that the sperm had been obtained illegally (i.e. without his written informed consent) and therefore could not be used, but the public sympathy for her plight was, I contend, a significant aspect of the eventual decision that allowed her to 'export' and hence use (successfully!) the sperm outside the jurisdiction of the UK Act.

Significantly, NE is now intractably infertile, and her only chance of a child to which she is genetically related lies with using these six embryos. LH is, by contrast, subfertile, but had or has the prospect of achieving a genetically related pregnancy either with a new partner or by using donor sperm.

In the case of NE, the couple were aware that their single cycle of IVF represented her only opportunity to become a biological mother. It is open to debate how informed either of the couple were about the possibility of using donor sperm to create embryos with NE's eggs, or that the Act effectively gave 'power of veto' over the use of their embryos to HJ.

The case of *McFall* vs. *Shimp* (1978)[3] may cast some light on the issue here. A man was found to be the only person with compatible bone marrow to save his cousin's life. After some reflection, the first cousin declined to have the tissue removed, even in the knowledge that his cousin would probably die as a result. The issue went to court, and the court, unsurprisingly, was unwilling to order the operation to harvest the bone marrow, even though the cousin's moral culpability was criticized heavily.

For LH and WH, they were aware that with 2 years' infertility as a couple, their best, but not their only, chance of parenthood lay with IVF. The fact that LH already has a biological child is of only marginal medical relevance, but seems to have had a significant (negative) influence on public opinion.

Modern fertility techniques, including cryopreservation of gametes and embryos, have permitted a temporal as well as a spatial separation to emerge between the existence of a relationship and the initiation of a pregnancy. It is no longer necessary to be 'together' or even alive to become biological parents. This has to a large extent ameliorated the asymmetry that has historically existed between men and women in the matter of conception.

Once a man had impregnated a woman (or otherwise given her access to a sample of his semen), there was nothing (legally) he could do about the resulting pregnancy if any. This was the case even if he had believed that she was using effective contraception (as in the celebrated US case of the man who sued his ex-girlfriend who had claimed to be taking the oral contraceptive pill – unsuccessfully – for 'sperm stealing'), or even if he had not been aware of the risk he was running (as Boris Becker found to his cost in a closet).

Once embryos have been created, however (and here we are not concerned with the moral status of the human embryo, or the point at which life may be said to begin, but simply that in at least 20% of favorable cases there is a realistic prospect of a healthy pregnancy and birth resulting from the transfer of frozen–thawed embryos), this historical asymmetry between men (who lose all power of veto at the point of ejaculation) and women (who enjoy absolute rights to control every aspect of the pregnancy including its destruction) no longer exists.

If we define 'power of consent' as the right to use the embryo with the consent of only one gamete provider and 'power of veto' as the right of either to prevent transfer or even continued storage, then we can envisage several possible scenarios in which the inherent symmetry/asymmetry of the reproductive relationship may be recognized, enshrined in law or overruled.

(In the interest of simplicity we must ignore the fact that, under the terms of the UK HFE Act, an embryo that is created using donor sperm for a woman in a relationship with a man who will be the 'social' and hence 'legal' father of any resulting child has theoretically the chance of its transfer being 'vetoed' by more than one man. We could also imagine a nightmare scenario in which a married couple who have achieved successful pregnancies through IVF agreed to donate their surplus embryos and then subsequently divorce, with the ex-wife wanting to withdraw her consent to the donation as she wishes to use the embryos herself to have what would be full siblings of her existing children, and the ex-husband wanting to withdraw his consent to the donation so that the embryos could be perished!)

The great divergence in size between gametes contributed to the creation of an embryo, and the greater physical contribution that the woman usually (but not inevitably, as in the case of a surrogate pregnancy) makes, should not necessarily be arguments against maintaining that symmetry exists between the man and the woman, and that both could have the power of consent or of veto (but not both). One argument for symmetry is that both parties face the same potential consequences, i.e. genetic or biological parenthood, from decisions made concerning the use of the embryos, so they should be treated equally. It may be the case, in the era of the 'one-night stand', that many men are never aware that they *are* fathers in the genetic if not functional sense, and probably as many believe, falsely, that the paternities which are attributed to them are truly theirs. But that would hardly entitle a woman to have disputed embryos transferred to her womb against the express desire of the 'father', by simply promising never to reveal to him or let him find out whether any child had been born as a result of the transfer.

Some sperm donors have described considerable distress and trauma at the mere prospect that there are 'children' of theirs 'out there somewhere' that they will never know or even know about. This situation may become acute when the donor becomes an actual, functional father and is aware of the real conundrum of the 'nature versus nurture' debate at first hand, or worse still, finds that he is unable to become a father.

A parallel explanation has been advanced to account for the decline in the number of young women willing to 'egg share' since the ending of donor anonymity in the UK. To suspect that one is a 'genetic' parent is one thing, but to be potentially confronted with the evidence, even 18 years later, is something else. This is not, however, to ignore the real joy that many adopted people find in discovering their 'genetic' roots or that they have siblings or half-siblings that they never knew about. We must hope that similar positive outcomes arise from contacts between people who have 'genetic' if not 'birth' relationships.

In both cases outlined above, it is the female ex-partner who sought transfer of the embryos to herself. If true symmetry, with the power of consent, but not veto were to exist, then the man must also have the right to access the embryos and try for pregnancy using a surrogate. This case for symmetry was raised by the US case of the divorced couple *JB* vs. *MB* in 2001[4]. The couple had signed a contract specifying certain conditions under which their embryos could be perished. MB, the man, wished to access the embryos for use by his new partner as a surrogate, but the court concluded that contracts that would force a person to become a parent at a future date, when it was against their will at that date, would be against public policy.

I allude above to the arguments for asymmetry that arise from comparisons with natural conception. If a woman need not necessarily inform a man that he is to be a genetic father, or may choose to terminate a pregnancy without his consent or even knowledge, then the 'natural' order would seem to be highly asymmetrical. During an IVF cycle, the woman bears the brunt of the physical demands of the treatment, and this has been advanced as an argument for the maintenance of 'asymmetry of control' residing with the woman about the disposition of frozen embryos.

Two US cases which attempted to arbitrate conflicting claims over frozen embryos illustrate the power of the 'appeal to asymmetry' that has influenced thought in this field. In the celebrated case of *Davis* vs. *Davis* (1990)[5], a divorcing couple contested the 'custody' of seven frozen embryos. The trial judge declared that the embryos were 'children *in vitro*', and awarded them to Mrs Davis on the grounds that it was in the best interest of the embryos to survive, and the party offering to facilitate that should prevail. Two years later the decision was reversed on appeal, with the Tennessee Supreme Court ruling that embryos are not persons, but also that the party wanting to avoid reproduction should control disposition of the embryos unless the embryos represented the only possibility for parenthood for the other party.

In another divorce hearing, in the rather different jurisdiction of New York, Mrs Kass (*Kass* vs. *Kass* (1998))[6] attempted to gain control of frozen embryos left over from ten unsuccessful IVF attempts. The couple had signed a prior agreement that, in the event that they no longer wished to try for a pregnancy together, or that they could not agree on the fate of their embryos, then they would donate them for research. The ex-wife was awarded control of the embryos on the grounds that in a normal 'conception' the woman controls the fate of the embryos, and that should apply even if they were *in vitro* rather than *in vivo*. This ruling was overturned on appeal, and the donation for research was enforced.

In a further US case of *AZ* vs. *BZ* (1999)[7], the Massachusetts court's decision concurred with the argument that consent made prior to treatment is unenforceable. The couple had signed 'consent forms' indicating that in the case of marital separation the embryos were to be available to the wife for implantation. It was revealed that the wife filled in the blank areas describing this course of action after her husband had signed blank forms. The court stated that the agreement at issue was unenforceable because of a 'change in circumstances' during the 4 years between the last signed consent and the bringing of the case to court. The court offered the statement '. . . even had the husband and wife entered into an unambiguous agreement between themselves regarding the disposition of the frozen preembryos, we would not enforce an agreement that would compel one donor to become a parent against his or her will.'

This leads us to consider the status of contracts in relation to fertility treatment in general, and the disposition of frozen embryos in particular. The use of superovulatory drug regimens and the contribution that frozen–thawed embryos make to the cumulative pregnancy rate for IVF and intracytoplasmic sperm injection (ICSI) treatment have focused increasing attention on the potential for frozen embryos. At the point that the HFE Act was placed on the statute book, the live birth rate from frozen embryo transfers was dismal, and this probably accounted for the fact that embryos created from donor eggs could escape the 6 months' quarantine required for sperm, and be transferred 'fresh'. Now the chance of implantation of good-quality frozen embryos is approaching that of fresh ones, and for the increasing number of women undergoing assisted reproductive technologies (ART) in their late 30s, there is little doubt that they are more likely to achieve an IVF pregnancy with an embryo created and frozen when they were 37 than with a 'fresh' embryo created when they were 40.

Significantly, couples may come to view the status of their surplus embryos quite differently when they know the outcome of their 'fresh' cycle. Couples who have had a negative test following a fresh transfer often disregard any potential from their frozen embryos and choose to embark on a further fresh cycle rather than use them. Couples who have had a live birth from a fresh cycle take a quite different attitude to their frozen embryos, truly regarding them as 'possible children', and this is what makes it so difficult for them to contemplate allowing them to perish at expiry of the storage period, be donated for implantation or be given to research[8]. In the UK, clinics are encouraged to go to extraordinary lengths to contact couples who have time-expired embryos in store, and it is quite clear that many couples would much rather the clinics perished the embryos when the expiry date was reached rather than give them, the couple, the 'moral responsibility' for ordering their destruction.

It is one of the great ironies of IVF and ICSI that couples who are most likely to get babies from their fresh cycle are also most likely to get supernumerary good-quality embryos for cryopreservation, frozen embryos which, in turn, are most likely to become babies too.

This would suggest that 'contracts' which couples sign prior to or during IVF treatment about the eventual disposition of their frozen embryos are literally and ethically worthless. A recent study found that a significant proportion of couples who could be contacted had indeed changed their minds since signing the forms about their frozen embryos' fate[9]. Many commercial clinics seem to be more concerned that they may end up storing embryos for which they cannot contact the couple and collect an annual storage fee, or that they may be liable in the case of the cryobank or even the clinic failing, than they are about couples' current wishes not being enacted.

Under UK law in the field of ART, power of veto for both parties recognizes a fundamental right to prevent the conception of a child with their genetic component against their will. It may be the case that half of all natural pregnancies are conceived 'by accident', but, concerning the use of cryopreserved embryos, the decision to (try to) become a parent should be informed and deliberate. Passion, alcohol and loneliness may all account for inadvertent conceptions, but coercion is never acceptable. Consider the thought experiment in which the problems of human reproductive cloning have been solved. One would be rightly outraged to discover that follicular cells taken from a hair 'tweaked' from your head by a passing stranger had, via nuclear transfer technology, been turned into an embryo containing your entire genome that was currently gestating in an unknown womb somewhere!

Having given due emphasis to the rights of the embryo (to respect, to identity, to a quality-controlled environment, etc.) as outlined in the HFE Act, then is there a sense in which the embryo's 'right to have a chance of existence' could trump the power of veto of (one of) its progenitors? If embryos are to be accorded any 'rights to life', then if one gamete provider did not want the embryo transferred, the other could claim access to the embryos, utilizing a surrogate if necessary. In the extreme case where neither gamete provider wanted the embryos or they could not be contacted, the embryos could be made available for 'adoption'. This was the attitude taken by 200 women from the Italian town of Massa, who, on learning that UK law required the destruction of more than 3000 time-expired or untraceable embryos, offered a group 'prenatal adoption' in preference to what they clearly regarded as infanticide[10]. This is not so different a mind-set from that of the Bush administration, which has recently made federal funding available to facilitate 'known' embryo donation where the donating couple will 'choose' the birth parents of their embryos with the expectation that the resulting siblings from the two families will be brought up with full knowledge of, and access to, each other.

Current social mores may influence our judgments about the structure of families and the significance of genetic links. Currently, one in five newborn babies leave the maternity ward to go home with their mother to an environment where there is no (related or unrelated) 'father'. One in four children in the UK grow up in a household in which they are not genetically linked to the 'father' figure (if any). Some 14% of babies do not have a father's name entered on their birth certificate. As social trends toward delayed motherhood and the developing pattern of 'serial' partnerships results in women endeavoring to conceive at older ages, age-related subfertility is an increasing cause of referral for fertility treatment. A recent survey found that only half of a large sample of childless women who had expressed a desire for children when surveyed in their early 30s *and* were in a position to try for pregnancy had actually become mothers when the survey was repeated in their late 30s. The average number of babies born per woman in Europe is now only 1.5: below 'replacement' level.

These sociological facts, however, cannot provide ethical direction. Article 8 of the Human Rights Act may 'protect the right to family life'[11], but it does not grant an entitlement to whatever fertility treatment is necessary to become a parent, even if this were to be technically feasible! It remains the case that forcing someone to become a (genetic) parent against their will is inevitably a more serious breach of rights than withholding treatment by refusing access to disputed embryos. Difficult cases, such as that of NE, where disputed embryos may represent the only chance of (genetic) and ordinary motherhood, may be considered to be so exceptional that different rules could apply.

This seems to be the position in the review of the *Davis* vs. *Davis* case by the US Supreme Court in 1992. Within their conclusion, they point to assessing the advantages and disadvantages for each of the gamete providers in order to reach a decision. 'If no prior agreement exists, then the relative interests of the parties in using or not using the preembryos must be weighed. Ordinarily, the party wishing to avoid procreation should prevail, assuming that the other party has a reasonable possibility of achieving parenthood by means other than the use of the preembryos in question. If no other reasonable alternatives exist, then the argument in favor of using the preembryos to achieve pregnancy should be considered.'

This seems terribly compassionate, but totally impractical, as it requires an inherently uncertain knowledge of an individual's fertility prospects. In the case of NE, where surgery has rendered impossible the prospect of any other embryos being created which are genetically related to her, this might constitute an 'exceptional case' as envisaged by the Supreme Court. Egg or embryo donation could in theory offer NE the chance of motherhood without compromise of HJ's legal rights.

Some might claim that HJ is more in the position of the cousin that could have been a bone-marrow donor, but chose not to because of the discomfort involved.

In other cultures, where 'collective parenting' is the norm, or in other times, such as in Victorian England, where 'child gifting' was seen as the obvious solution to unmatched demand and supply of children within extended families, the assumption that knowledge of the source of someone's genes defines their place in society would be questioned. As DNA fingerprinting increasingly reveals that some of us are not (genetically) who we think are, and 'alternative' family structures are increasingly represented in society, an opportunity is provided for the ART community and society at large to consider the 'ethical' as opposed to the 'scientific' significance of a little bundle of cells not quite visible to the naked eye.

REFERENCES

1. Re F (in utero) [1998] 2 All ER 193.
2. Human Fertilisation and Embryology Act 1990. www.hfea.gov.uk.
3. McFall vs. Shimp (1978) 10Pa D and C 3d 90.
4. JB vs. MB WL 909294 [2001].
5. Davis vs. Davis 842 SW 2d 588, 597 [Tenn 1992].
6. Kass vs. Kass 696 NE 2d 174 [NY 1998].
7. AZ vs. BZ 431 Mass 150 [1999].
8. Kovacs G, Breheny S, Dear M. Embryo donation at an Australian university in-vitro fertilisation clinic: issues and outcomes. Med J Aust 2003; 178: 127–9.
9. Klock SC, Sheinin S, Kazer RR. The disposition of unused frozen embryos. N Engl J Med 2001; 345: 69–70.
10. Demartis F. Mass pre-embryo adoption. Camb Q Healthcare Ethics 1998; 7: 101–3.
11. Human Rights Act. www.YourRights.org.uk.

Chapter 2

Human cloning: reproductive crime or therapeutic panacea – where are we now?

Françoise Shenfield, Charles Babinet and Gérard Teboul

Human cloning; reproductive (crime?) and therapeutic (panacea?)

Warning: The following must be read within the context of events which occurred in the last week of 2005 and the first week of 2006, when the Korean researcher Hwang, admitted falsification of his findings (published as reference 11). The hopes of patients and scientists have been brutally dashed or at least seriously challenged by this breach of trust which results from the fundamental ethical assault on the principle of truth telling, without which our autonomy is not respected as we cannot obtain proper information, one of its enabling tools. At a time when earlier work (see reference 2) is under investigation, introspection is the order of the day, for the scientific as well as the lay press, and for any honest citizen whose enthusiasm for good news in the perennial fight against disease has perhaps lessened their critical appraisal ability.

The term 'cloning' first captured public imagination in 1997 with publication of the method of somatic cell nuclear transfer (SCNT) which led to the birth of Dolly[1]. Although this example was highlighted worldwide as a danger to humanity as we know it, few adversaries to the employment of human embryos for therapeutic research now use this fear of application to reproductive human cloning as an argument against proceeding with therapeutic stem-cell research. As described in the legal section of this chapter, several international declarations and national legislations have clearly forbidden this unsafe technique. The possibilities of using embryonic stem cells for therapy, and the first successful SCNT in the human embryo, described in Korea in 2004, renewed hopes for the eventual use of human embryos for therapy of serious diseases[2], and have largely overshadowed the debates on reproductive cloning of the late 1990s.

This does not mean that reproductive cloning has completely disappeared from the headlines or that politicians have let the subject rest as not worthy of their attention. Indeed, last year President Chirac suggested that it should be deemed 'a crime against the human person', a term of indictment which differs from that of 'crime against humanity', as this would be unacceptable terminology, reserved as it is for events of large-scale horror which were only too frequent in the last century. Strong words, however, reflect strong feelings reflected by battles in the European Parliament and at the United Nations (UN). Public understanding has grown, the different issues raised by therapeutic cloning and the use of embryonic stem cells have been the subject of many articles and many US citizens have voted on the subject at the occasion of the recent presidential elections.

It is therefore appropriate to ask 'Where are we now?', considering the facts as applied to human cloning, the complex legislative background in the growing field of international law and the ethical issues involved in both reproductive and therapeutic cloning. The facts are a basis for our analysis, but ethical and legal issues somewhat overlap, as the law tries to encapsulate many of the moral issues, albeit influenced by diverse social and historical backgrounds.

THE FACTS

The cloning of various mammalian species and increased knowledge of stem cell biology have both attracted considerable interest from the scientific community and in the public domain in recent years[3,4]. This is due not only to scientific interest in basic research – understanding how mammalian organisms develop – but also to the potential use of stem cells to devise protocols to cure various human diseases, e.g. Parkinson's and neurodegenerative diseases, diabetes or myocardial infarction. The general idea is to take advantage of the unique properties of stem cells, which have the ability both to self-renew and to give rise to differentiated cells of various types, depending on the particular stem cell considered and the experimental conditions used for inducing their differentiation. Such properties of stem cells could be used to produce the appropriate differentiated cells and transfer them to a patient, in the hope that they regenerate damaged or diseased tissue. This approach is therefore called 'cell replacement therapy', and has, in fact, long been used in bone marrow transfer to replace leukemic blood cells, based on the well-characterized existence in the bone marrow of hematopoietic stem cells able to differentiate in the various cell types present in the blood (red cells, lymphocytes, etc.).

Stem cells may be classified by their differentiation potential as pluripotent, multipotent, oligopotent and unipotent, that is, giving rise to many, several, few or a single cell type, respectively. This short overview concentrates on the most versatile stem cells, called embryonic stem (ES) cells, with a view to explain how the fascinating properties of these particular stem cells, in combination with embryo cloning, could pave the way in the long term to the use of cell replacement therapy in the human.

ES cells were first isolated more than 20 years ago from cultured mouse embryos as blastocysts. It was soon demonstrated, by introducing a few of these cells in a young host embryo, that they had the ability to contribute to all the tissues of the embryo, including its germline. Furthermore, ES cells can be maintained indefinitely in culture while retaining their developmental properties.

In addition, it was demonstrated that it was possible to orientate their differentiation *in vitro* and, under specific conditions, toward particular cell lineage such as neurons, muscle, skin, adipose tissue, etc.[5]. It should be mentioned that, in recent years, such protocols directing the differentiation of mouse ES cells in culture toward a particular cell type have been much improved, so that it is now possible to obtain almost pure populations of differentiated cells. This is the case, for example, for some types of neurons which can be used in a cell therapy protocol to repopulate the brain of mice deficient in these neurons[6].

ES cells having properties similar to mouse ES cells were isolated in 1998 from human blastocysts, donated by couples following *in vitro* fertilization, and since then several groups worldwide have isolated many new human ES (hES) cell lines[7]. Although it was not possible, for obvious reasons, to evaluate their *in vivo* contribution to embryonic development, it was shown in culture that they could be induced, like mouse ES cells, to differentiate into numerous cell types. Moreover and most important, these hES cells retain their stem cell properties, even after prolonged culture (more than 100 cell doublings). However, the potential use of hES cells for cell replacement therapy raises, among many others, one obvious issue: immune rejection must be avoided. Thus, ideally, cells destined to be used for cell replacement therapy should come from the patient him-/herself. In this case, they would be genetically identical, and therefore not subject to immune rejection. To solve this problem, one possibility would be to take advantage of the properties of embryos obtained by SCNT and of hES cells (SCNT-hES) thereof derived. As is now well known, it has been possible to 'clone' different mammalian species, including sheep (Dolly), but also mice, pigs, bovines and, more recently, rabbits, rats, cats and horses. This is done by introducing a nucleus from a differentiated cell into an enucleated oocyte, culturing this manipulated oocyte for a short period to obtain a 'nuclear transfer' embryo at blastocyst stage and then implanting it into a foster mother to allow development to term, giving rise to a 'clone', i.e. an organism having the same genetic make-up as the one from which the nucleus has been taken. Those results have been spectacular, and demonstrate that the oocyte cytoplasm may 'reprogram' the incoming adult nucleus into an embryonic nucleus. However, the underlying mechanism of reprogramming is obscure and probably inadequate in most cases, resulting in the poor efficiency of cloning: only around 1% of nuclear-transfer embryos are born, and the clones born, in many instances, exhibit various anomalies[4,8]. In the context of cell replacement therapy, however, blastocysts may be put into culture to try and derive 'SCNT-ES' cells, using the same methodology as for blastocysts obtained by fertilization. These SCNT-hES cells could then be used to obtain the appropriate differentiated cells for cell replacement therapy. The whole procedure, at variance with reproductive cloning described above, is usually called 'therapeutic cloning'. In fact, such a scenario has been followed in the mouse model and indicated that it was possible to derive cell lines with properties of ES cells from nuclear-transfer blastocysts (NT-ES cells)[9]; such cells have been used for cell replacement therapy to treat mouse models of an immunodeficiency[10] and Parkinson's disease[6].

In 2004, a Korean team presented, for the first time, evidence of the isolation of human nuclear-transfer ES cells (NT-hES) from a cloned blastocyst, but with poor efficiency[2]. However, remarkably, the same team published a new study in May 2005, with impressive rates of success[11]. Indeed, using the transfer of skin fibroblasts into an enucleated oocyte, they were able to isolate with high efficiency, 11 NT-hES cell lines, from patients who had a genetic immunodeficiency disease, or spinal cord injury, or juvenile diabetes, all of which could potentially be treated by cell replacement therapy.

Several criteria were used to ascertain the nature and genetic origin of the NT-hES line. Indeed, these cells expressed different markers specific to ES cells, and they had a normal karyotype. They were also shown to have the ability to differentiate into derivatives of the three embryonic germ-cell layers. Finally, and most important, their genetic make-up was shown to be the very one predicted from the nuclear donor. The logical follow-up of this study will be to devise efficient ways of coaxing NT-hES cells to differentiate in the appropriate cell types, depending on the disease, and implant these cells in the patient. Obviously, the results of this study indicate that the researchers in this Korean team have been able to improve greatly the efficiency of NT-hES cell isolation by changing aspects of the protocol, but also probably by improving their skill. There is no doubt that this study represents a milestone on the long road to cell replacement therapy. Furthermore, it is important to note that the availability of NT-hES cells derived from diseased people should be a precious asset in understanding the mechanisms underlying the development of the disease[12].

Altogether, results obtained in the mouse model and the recent and very significant success in isolating NT-hES from different patients, suggest that therapeutic cloning could become a reality. This may take a long time, as several issues need to be addressed and problems solved. Among them are, notably, a more extensive analysis of the normality of NT-hES cells (for example their imprinting status[2]), and devising efficient ways of deriving pure populations of the relevant differentiated cells, in particular devoid of contaminating ES cells which have a high tumorigenic potential when implanted in ectopic sites. At the same time, it will be very important to test the functionality of the differentiated cells, i.e. their ability to play their physiological role in the *in vivo* environment.

LEGAL ASPECTS

From a legal perspective, it is not surprising that there is a consensus of opinion with regard to reproductive cloning (it is, generally speaking, rejected), and that therapeutic cloning is accompanied by sometimes bitter intellectual debates resulting in division. It is clear to see that it is the *finality* of cloning (is its purpose to cure or to reproduce?), rather than the *technology per se* required to perform it, which may give rise to different reactions.

In this context, the jurist is led to suggest that legislation takes into consideration the consequences engendered by research into the area of cloning. With regard to reproductive cloning, there is one danger in particular that must be taken into account: that of the (very probable) malformation of children arising from an embryo created following a nucleus transfer. It is therefore necessary to envisage legislation banning it (at least on a temporary basis). However, this legislation targets an aspect of living science of which researchers have no real knowledge: on a practical level (and, at least, officially) a child has not yet been born by means of cloning. Thus, in the case in point, the jurist who expresses that he is in favor of the existence of a prohibitive standard is acting in anticipation; on that score, *the rule of law precedes science*. In this respect, we find ourselves at the very opposite pole to the process that frequently characterizes creation of the laws of bioethics: these latter are often revised to take evolutions in science into account; in other words, *science precedes the rule of law* because, in the field of bioethics, the legislator contents himself with intervening to harmonize the legal standard with the new scientific techniques being offered to the public. Indeed, with regard to the sampling of hematopoietic stem cells and domino transplants, the Conseil d'Etat (French council of state) report, relative to revision of the bioethical laws of 1994, stated: 'Certain sampling techniques, developed since 1994, fall *de facto* outside the current legal framework . . . *It is necessary to adapt the texts to the evolution of the techniques . . .*'[13].

Within the international community, it may be observed that cloning has been the subject of numerous discussions which have been expressed in the form of a variety of texts: individual statements on the part of states[14], communiqués emanating from several states[15], positions of principle adopted by non-governmental organizations (NGOs)[16], resolutions and declarations emanating from international governmental organizations (IGOs)[17,18], international convention proposals[18] and even the existence of a treaty[19].

First, we should put human cloning within the context of conventional international law, and analyze the UN and the draft universal convention against human cloning.

Drawing up, within the framework of the UN, a universal convention against human cloning did not pose any particular difficulties at first analysis. In 2001, the fight led by France and Germany – who requested that the agenda of the United Nations General Assembly include a point of order entitled: 'International convention against the cloning of human beings for reproductive purposes'[20] – gained extensive support.

The objective sought by the Franco-German alliance was the following: to oppose the launch of the first international program for human cloning for reproductive purposes[21].

The Franco-German project was very soon rivaled by another project with the backing, in particular, of Spain, the USA and Italy. This project proposed the prohibition, within one and the same instrument, of reproductive *and* therapeutic cloning[22]. Henceforth, the member states of the UN were divided, and this division led to the stagnation of the original project.

Paradoxically, the desire to ban cloning completely (reproductive *and* therapeutic) served the interests of those favorable to reproductive cloning. From the moment that negotiations in this domain reached stalemate, no international texts of a binding nature were adopted, and, consequently, there was no legal prohibition of a conventional nature in existence.

Nevertheless, in late December 2004, the General Assembly of the United Nations decided to create a working group to finalize, using a draft resolution originating from Italy[23], the text of a United Nations declaration on human cloning. Approximately two and a half months later, the General Assembly adopted a definitive text, differing from the Italian draft resolution, notably stating that member states of the UN 'are called upon to prohibit all forms of human cloning inasmuch as they are incompatible with human dignity and the protection of human life'[24]. But the United Nations declaration on human cloning did not receive the unanimous support of the General Assembly: although it received 84 votes in its favor, there were 34 oppositions, along with 37 abstentions[25].

It can thus be seen that the shift from a conventional instrument, which was the initial aim, to a declaratory instrument did not contribute to eliminate entirely differences of opinion between states. Significantly, it would come to light that certain states in favor of therapeutic cloning had voted against this declaration. This was notably the case of the United Kingdom, which highlighted, by means of its representative, the existence of the risk that the declaration could be interpreted in such a way as to constitute 'a call for a total ban on all forms of human cloning'[26]. It should also be stressed that France has not expressed any opposition to international attempts at therapeutic cloning, even though it has prohibited this form of cloning on its own territory[27] by a law voted in in 2004, at the risk of penalties. However, research on stem cells issued from supernumerary embryos is now permitted in France by that very same law.

At the European level, we may look at the first Protocol to the Oviedo Convention on the prohibition of cloning human beings; 'open for signature' on 4 April 1997, the convention on human rights and biomedicine[28] (known as the Oviedo Convention) does not contain any provision explicitly banning human cloning. However, the first Protocol to the Oviedo Convention, executed in Paris on 12 January 1998, expressly prohibits reproductive cloning. Its first article §1 states that 'Any intervention seeking to create a human being genetically identical to another human being, whether living or dead, is prohibited'. It should be noted that this regulation lays down a general and absolute prohibition: 'general' because 'any intervention' is banned; in other words, any cloning technique – irrespective of whether it involves blastomere separation or nucleus transfer – is outlawed under the first article §1 of the Paris Protocol; 'absolute' because article 2 of the same protocol states that 'no derogation from the provisions of this Protocol shall be made under article 26, paragraph 1, of the Convention'. In other words, the prohibition standard set out in article 1§1 may not be subject to any restriction.

It should be added that the authors of the first Protocol demonstrated a laudable pragmatism. From a scientific perspective, 'a human being genetically identical to another human being' is, in the strict sense of the phrase, a human being, *all* of whose genes (whether they are nuclear or otherwise) are identical. However, article 1§2 of the Paris Protocol states that 'the term human being "genetically identical" to another human being means a human being sharing with another the same nuclear gene set'. Therefore, in the sense of article 1§2 of the Protocol of 1998, two human beings who have the same nuclear genes but whose mitochondrial genes are dissimilar have the status of a clone.

But what is the situation with regard to therapeutic cloning? In this domain, the concept of a 'human being' is of the utmost importance. Should a distinction be made between a 'human being' and a 'human person'? The first article of the Oviedo convention calls for a difference to be made between the idea of a 'human being' and the idea of a 'person'. In this respect, it may be considered that the term 'human being' refers not only to an individual who has already been born, but also to an individual in the process of being created, from the initial stage of him/her conception; under this reasoning the original zygote would be termed a 'human being'. However, '*it was decided to leave it to domestic law to define the scope of the expression 'human being'* for the purposes of the application of the present [first] Protocol'[29]. In this regard, it may be noted that The Netherlands, in a declaration recognized by specialists and submitted to the Secretary General of the Council of Europe, stated that 'In relation to Article 1 of the Protocol, the Government of the Kingdom of the Netherlands declares that it interprets the term 'human being' as referring exclusively to a human individual, i.e. a human being who has been born'. It thus would appear that the first Protocol to the Oviedo Convention does not *objectively* prohibit therapeutic cloning.

It should be added that, in virtue of article 33 of the Oviedo Convention (and article 4 of its first Protocol), five states, who are not members of the Council of Europe, may consent to be bound by these two international agreements. These states, whose importance in terms of bioethics is not inconsiderable, are the following: Australia, Canada, the United States, Japan and the Holy See. Moreover, the Oviedo Convention and the first Protocol thereto have vocation to universal authority. However, in practical terms this authority remains without effect: no state (that is not a member of the Council of Europe) is bound – on the date on which this article was written – by the Convention of 1997 and by the Protocol of 1998. There are, however, several instances of national laws which ban reproductive cloning (UK, Belgium, Greece[30-32]), a direct reflection of the generalized reprobation following the much publicized 'attempts' at the method. Below follows an analysis of the background in ethical terms to this practically international revulsion, and of the dilemmas of 'therapeutic cloning'.

ETHICAL ISSUES

In the articles and comments (mostly) condemning reproductive cloning, words such as dignity, identity, sameness and the moral sense of 'self' have been analyzed at length, notwithstanding the fact that the technique is far from safe, which provides the main and overwhelming objection. One may also object on the grounds that reproductive cloning would threaten the autonomy of the future cloned person, who may be treated by society as somewhat predetermined, entailing as it does an increase in (genetic) determinism even if relative, as the clone is born into another environment than the person replicated. This, and the psychological arguments, seem to be the only worthwhile arguments opposing the proponents of reproductive cloning: the narcissistic venture of the parent(s) may well threaten the building of the identity of the child, mostly by decreasing the possibility of separation from the initial model and thus his/her autonomy. This is coupled with the danger of instrumentalization by either one person or a group of other persons and the danger of eugenics (European Group on Ethics in Science and New Technologies, EGE[33]).

It is with this in mind that the European Society of Human Reproduction and Embryology (ESHRE) issued a statement 'to continue the ban on reproductive cloning', after a 5-year voluntary moratorium on reproductive cloning in 1999 when it became clear that technical advances arising from cloning animals could theoretically result in an attempt to clone a human. This happened in January 2003, after Clonaid's claim that the first human clone had been born, when ESHRE's Executive Committee stated that its moratorium would continue, and dissociated the organization from any attempts at human reproductive cloning. It also stated that it was important that the whole field of stem cell research and therapeutic cloning was not damaged by being caught up in the outcry over reproductive cloning.

Fortunately, the repulsion caused almost universally by reproductive cloning has not been universally matched by the same feelings or arguments about the use of stem cells from human embryos. Britain was the first state to allow therapeutic cloning. Embryo research has been licensed under strict conditions since the Human Fertilisation and Embryology (HFE) Act 1990[34], permitting only research linked to reproduction. After a democratic process involving a report by the Chief Medical Officer[35] and a vote in both chambers of the Houses of Parliament, new categories were added to Statute 31 Jan 2001[30], allowing, this time, 'research for serious disease'. Interestingly, a 'pro-life' lobby has asked a judge[36] to assess whether an embryo created by SCNT would actually qualify to be such an entity in terms of the HFE Act 1990. Whatever our leanings, whether more deontological or utilitarian, most agents involved in the debate would probably agree that honesty is a virtue not to be sacrificed. It seems, therefore, honest to say that an embryo is an embryo whatever way it was created and even if not replaced into the uterus. Finally, the Court of Appeal said that a cloned embryo did fall within the legal definition of an embryo. The judges argued that the spirit of the law was intended to include cloned embryos. Lord Phillips added: 'If Parliament had known of the cloning technique in 1990 it would certainly have been included in the legislation which controls research and use of embryos'.

Another approach is that, of the Infertility Treatment Authority in the state of Victoria, Australia[37], which stated that 'ES cells . . . are not the equivalent of an intact embryo . . . as a clump of ES cells transferred to a uterus would not become a viable fetus'. As the Victoria Act[38] forbids destructive research on embryos, it means that in this case the definition of an embryo according to the Act does not apply to ES cells, and research therefore not illegal in Victoria. But this is different from stating that the embryo, before its blastocyst stage and potential stem cells, does not deserve its name if created a certain way, as by SCNT.

Aware of the potential exploitation of these semantic games[39], an ESHRE Taskforce[40] defined the preimplantation embryo in its first ethics consideration on behalf of the society. The Taskforce stressed that this term was descriptive, meaning the embryo out of the body before it is given a chance of becoming a fetus and then a legal person by means of embryo transfer. But such a descriptive term does not imply a lesser quality. We, practitioners and scientists, should not use semantic particulars which would allow opponents to any kind of research to deride professionals who might simply rename the entity 'embryo' in order to make the consequences of its use more acceptable. The difficulties outlined here are illustrated by the many different national legal definitions[41] of the embryo for statutory purposes, whilst there is usually no definition of the beginning of life. At international level, declarations often use symbolic language, which complicates matters even further, as it is extremely difficult to reconcile the pragmatic and the symbolic.

Meanwhile, specific issues arise from the possible application of animal stem-cell research to the human embryo. With this in mind, the ESHRE Taskforce on Law and Ethics considered the matter of stem cell technology[42]. Essential to the analysis is the definition of a stem cell: a cell which retains the ability to self-renew and to differentiate into one or several cell types. Stem cells may be derived from the embryo, the fetus or the adult, but our purpose in this chapter dedicated to 'cloning' is to concentrate on the ethical issues related to embryonic stem (ES) cells derived from the blastocyst.

Many fundamental ethical questions in this field are far from new. Indeed, consent must be obtained for research, reflecting the principle of autonomy. But the Taskforce stresses that 'in view of the special nature of stem cells and their longevity, it should be specifically mentioned that the embryos will be used for research into the establishment of cell lines which can be kept indefinitely, may eventually be used for therapeutic purposes, and will never be replaced into a uterus'. It should also be made clear whether the cells may be used for commercial and/or clinical purposes. This is therefore specific rather than general consent.

There are also specific ethical considerations according to the source of cells, and especially regarding the creation of embryos specifically for research. The

ESHRE Taskforce's first consideration on ethics and law for the preimplantation embryo states: 'we do not object to embryo research on supernumerary embryos nor do we find any major ethical differences with embryos created for research within (specific) constraints. The constraint imposed is essential however: the creation and the possibility of research on pre implantation embryos specifically created for the purpose is appropriate only if the information cannot be obtained by research on supernumerary zygotes'. Indeed, this issue of the creation of embryos for research is especially vexing. Whilst article 18 of the European Convention on Human Rights and Biomedicine[28] specifically forbids this, in the UK the Human Fertilisation and Embryology Authority (HFEA) is charged with overseeing embryo research within limits according to a licensing system: the creation of embryos *de novo* for research is not unlawful, but its 'necessity' must be demonstrated, ensuring that embryos are not created for futile reasons.

Other issues are also of grave concern. For instance, the question of patenting evokes a number of ethical and legal questions. This proposed declaration of the Taskforce wishes to emphasize that the patenting policy should not hamper the development of new technologies or slow down the acquisition of knowledge. Given the huge potential benefits for a considerable number of patients suffering from various diseases, the health of the population in general should take priority over commercial goals. Moreover, patenting should not unduly restrict the fundamental principle of 'freedom of research'.

However, in practice, the specific issue of the source of oocytes used for any embryos created for the purpose of research is a major problem, in view of the already well-documented imbalance between need and supply in the case of egg donation. As there are a limited number of oocytes available, should they preferentially be allocated to reproduction? The potential abuse of vulnerable women who might be enticed to sell their oocytes for research is certainly a grave concern, as it has been for several years in the field of gamete donation.

At European level, though, the EGE[43] has been more conservative in its recommendations, made public last November. The commission stresses again, in its final report, the Charter of fundamental rights of the European Union approved by the European Council in Biarritz in October 2000, that reproductive cloning is forbidden.

The EGE deems ethically unacceptable the creation of embryos from donated gametes, because supernumerary embryos are an alternative available source; in the case of embryos obtained by SCNT, it voices its extreme concern, whilst aware that 'the creation of [such] embryos may be the most effective way of obtaining pluripotent stem cells genetically identical to the patient and thus obtaining perfectly compatible tissues with the aim of avoiding rejection after transplantation'. The prime objection concerns the danger of exploiting women donors: 'these remote therapeutic perspectives must be balanced . . . with the risks of the use of embryos trivialisation, and of exerting pressure on women as sources of oocytes, and increasing the possibility of their instrumentalisation'. It finally considers that it applies the principle of proportionality by adopting a precautionary approach, and itself qualifies its own approach by the word 'prudence', taking into account that '[there is already] a vast field of research to explore with the other sources of stem cells'.

Finally, the EGE also recommends that EU funding should be made available, within the usual frame of research, and also tackles the concerns in research in this field. Specifically it mentions: 'the free and informed consent of donors and of recipients, and of the possible use of the embryo cells for the specific purpose in question'; and 'the need to protect anonymity of donors, whilst (retaining) traceability of donors and recipients in case unsatisfactory side-effects occur'.

Thus we may conclude that many consider stem cells from embryos created by SCNT a feminist issue, because the main danger lies in the exploitation of women, enticing them to relinquish oocytes by coercion. This is a fair comment at a time where the disproportion between donation of and demand for oocytes is prevalent everywhere, although this objection may be rethought if/when *in vitro* maturation becomes a better source of oocytes. Thus, the compromise 'wait and see' attitude of the EGE may be regarded as wise, or as lacking vision, but it certainly addresses all the issues in depth. Nevertheless, scientists in the field agree that research should continue with all sources of stem cells, as we cannot know now which source is going to fulfill the therapeutic promise, if any. All over the world, legislation, declaration and recent rapid advances in research into animal and human embryonic cloning with or without SCNT have ensured that the debate is evidence based[44], and both alive and lively[45]. That ethics and politics are interrelated, in the spirit of Aristotle's statement that to be a moral person is to act as a citizen in the city, has never been more aptly illustrated than by the great cloning debate[46]. It beholds us all, scientists or not, to take part in this informed debate, and reflect, so that beneficence is achieved and justice upheld without discrimination against the vulnerable or the poor.

That women are more vulnerable than men the world over, and students than teachers, either pre- or postgraduate, has sadly only very recently been illustrated by the sudden resignation of the leader of the team whose achievement made cloning history very recently[2,11]. The media had a field day, scientists' and ethicists' hearts sank, and perhaps the whole field had a setback when it transpired that oocytes were obtained under what could arguably be called psychological duress, therefore negating the principle of free, informed consent and the respect of the autonomy of the concerned (female) subject[47]. This event confirms that one may call therapeutic cloning a feminist (or women's reproductive rights) issue, as long as the source of oocytes is a woman, and not a tissue, or indeed a cloned gamete as may happen in the future.

REFERENCES

1. Wilmut I, Schnieke AE, McWhir J, et al. Viable offspring derived from fetal and adult mammary cells. Nature 1997; 387: 810–13.

2. Hwang WS, Ryu YJ, Park JH, et al. Evidence of a pluripotent human embryonic stem cell line derived from a cloned blastocyst. Science 2004; 303: 1669–74.

3. Lovell-Badge R. The future for stem cell research. Nature 2001; 414: 88–91.

4. Solter D. Mammalian cloning: advances and limitations. Nat Rev Genet 2000; 1: 199–207.

5. Nichols J. Introducing embryonic stem cells. Curr Biol 2001; 11: R503–5.

6. Barberi T, Klivenyi P, Calingasan NY, et al. Neural subtype specification of fertilization and nuclear transfer embryonic stem cells and application in parkinsonian mice. Nat Biotechnol 2003; 21: 1200–7.

7. Cowan CA, Klimanskaya I, McMahon J, et al. Derivation of embryonic stem-cell lines from human blastocysts. N Engl J Med 2004; 350: 1353–6.

8. Jaenisch R. Human cloning – the science and ethics of nuclear transplantation. N Engl J Med 2004; 351: 2787–91.

9. Wakayama T, Tabar V, Rodriguez I, et al. Differentiation of embryonic stem cell lines generated from adult somatic cells by nuclear transfer. Science 2001; 292: 740–3.

10. Rideout WM 3rd, Hochedlinger K, Kyba M, et al. Correction of a genetic defect by nuclear transplantation and combined cell and gene therapy. Cell 2002; 109: 17–27.

11. Hwang WS, Roh SI, Lee BC, et al. Patient-specific embryonic stem cells derived from human SCNT blastocysts. Science 2005; 308: 1777–83.

12. Pera MF, Trounson AO. Human embryonic stem cells: prospects for development. Development 2004; 131: 5515–25.

13. Conseil d'Etat, Les lois de bioéthique: cinq ans après. Les études du Conseil d'Etat. Paris: La Documentation française, 1999: 78.

14. Verbal note dated 17 October 2003, sent to the Office of Legal Affairs of the United Nations Secretariat by the Permanent Mission of Cuba to the United Nations. A/C.6/58/L.15, 17 October 2003.

15. G8 communiqué. Denver summit, 22 June 1997: §47.

16. International Federation of Gynaecology and Obstetrics (FIGO). Ethical guidelines regarding cloning (Cairo, March 1998). Gynecol Obstet Invest 1999; 48: 75–6.

17. Resolution of 12 March 1997, the European Parliament, and article 11 of the Universal declaration on the human genome, adopted by the UNESCO general conference, 11 November 1997.

18. Draft international convention for the prohibition of human cloning in all forms, put forward by Costa Rica. A/58/73, 17 April 2003: 2–10.

19. First Protocol to the Oviedo Convention forbidding cloning. Treaty Office, January 1998. www.coe.int.

20. United Nations. General Assembly. A/56/192, 7 August 2001: 1. www.un.org.

21. Le premier projet de clonage reproductif humain unanimement condamné [The first human reproductive cloning project universally condemned]. Le Monde, 9 August 2001: 5.

22. Teboul G. Un instrument international prohibant le clonage humain reproductif [An international instrument prohibiting human reproductive cloning]? Int J Bioethics 2004; 15: 85–93 (especially 88–89).

23. United Nations General Assembly. A/C.6/59/L.26*, 14 January 2005 (Italy: draft resolution) (cf. also United Nations General Assembly. A/C.6/59/L.27, 16 February 2005: 1§1.

24. United Nations General Assembly. United Nations Declaration on human cloning. A/RES/59/280, 23 March 2005: 2, point b/ of Declaration. (General Assembly approved, on 8 March 2005, United Nations Declaration on human cloning.).

25. Ad Hoc Committee on an International Convention against the Reproductive Cloning of Human Beings (and, more particularly, Activities undertaken in 2004/2005). www.un.org.

26. Jones Parry E. United Nations General Assembly, 82nd plenary session. A/59/PV 82, 8 March 2005: 4.

27. Loi no 2004-800 du 6 août 2004 relative a la bioethique. www.legifrance.gouv.fr.

28. Oviedo Convention. Treaty Office, 1997 www.coe.int.

29. Explanatory report of the Additional protocol to the Convention on human rights and biomedicine on the prohibition of cloning human beings: §6. Treaty Office. www.coe.int.

30. Human Reproductive Cloning Act 2001 (4 December 2001): 1. The offence. www.legislation.hmso.gov.uk/acts/acts2001/20010023.

31. Art. 6 de la loi du 11 mai 2003 (recherche sur les embryons in vitro). Moniteur belge, 28 mai 2003: 29288.

32. Art. 1 de la loi 3089/2002 (assistance médicale à la reproduction humaine) relatif, notamment, à l'article 1455 du Code civil grec. www.ciec-sg/Legislationpdf/Grèce.

33. European Commission. Opinion of the Group of Advisors on the Ethical Implications of Biotechnology to the European Commission: Ethical aspects of Cloning Techniques, rapporteur: Dr Anne McLaren, Brussels, 28 May 1997.

34. Human Fertilisation and Embryology Act 1990. London: HMSO, 1990

35. Stem cell research: medical progress with responsibility. London: Department of Health, June 2000. www.doh.gov.uk.

36. The Queen on the application of Pro-Life Alliance vs. Secretary of State for Health. High Court CO/4095/2000.

37. Infertility Treatment Authority. The use of embryonic stem cells. Victoria, Australia: ITA, 2000. www.ita.org.au.

38. Infertility Treatment Act 1995, State of Victoria, Australia.

39. Shenfield F. Semantics and ethics of human embryonic stem-cell research. Lancet 2005; 365: 2071–3.

40. ESHRE Taskforce on Law and Ethics I. The moral status of the pre-implantaion embryo. Hum Reprod 2001; 16: 1046–8.

41. IFFS Surveillance 04. Fertil Steril 2004; 81(Suppl 4): S9–54.

42. ESHRE. Ethical considerations: stem cells. 14 May 2001, wwww.eshre.com.

43. European Group on Ethics in Science and New Technologies to the European Commission. Adoption of an Opinion on Ethical Aspects of Human Cell Research and Use, Paris, 14 November 2000 (revised edition January 2001). Brussels: Secretariat of EGE 2001.

44. Vats A, Bielby RC, Tolley NS, et al. Stem cells. Lancet 2005; 366: 592–606.

45. Scolding N. Stem-cell therapy: hope and hype. Lancet 2005; 365: 2074–5.

46. Hopkings Tanne J. US president and Congress set to clash over stem cell research. Br Med J 2005; 330: 1285.

47. Parry J. Korean women rush to donate eggs after research pioneer resigns. Br Med J 2005; 331: 1291.

PART II

THE INTENDED PARENTS
AND FAMILY WELFARE

Chapter 3

Till death do us part: to be or not to be . . . a parent after one's death?

Gulam Bahadur

INTRODUCTION

This chapter draws on experiences gained in cases of posthumous reproduction, making use of legal studies and considering case reports to examine the motives of gestating women. It discusses the ethical considerations involved, and considers the legal and regulatory framework around assisted reproduction in the UK and in other countries.

Rapid innovations in reproductive technology, gamete retrieval and cryo-preservation have created new possibilities in human procreation, as a result of which new ethical and policy dilemmas have arisen. The issues raised by the topic of posthumous reproduction are some of the most challenging, difficult and sensitive that one is likely to encounter in any field of medicine, entailing complex moral, ethical and legal concerns.

It has become possible to retrieve, freeze and store sperm, embryos and even oocytes or ovarian tissue, thereby allowing new uses for this technology. Men and women who receive cancer therapy that will leave them sterile now have the option of storing gametes for use later in life. The rapid rate of technological advances means that new treatments are being rushed into use before they are proven safe or effective, potentially putting some women and children at risk of physical and psychological harm.

The death of a husband is a difficult time for a widow to make a rational decision about whether she wants the sperm of her dead husband to be harvested[1-3]. Because illnesses in the deceased partner are often unanticipated, the patient typically has not given prior consent for sperm retrieval. In these situations, physicians who are asked to perform sperm retrieval and storage face an array of difficult ethical issues. These include the question of whether posthumous reproduction is ethically justifiable, and whether it is ethical to retrieve spermatozoa from patients who are dead or in a persistent vegetative state (PVS). If retrieved spermatozoa are frozen, what should be the terms of the sperm storage agreement? Should there be time limits on storage? Should there be restrictions on the person who can be inseminated, or should the use of a surrogate be permitted? Additional dilemmas lie in the form of the legal requirements to have effective consent from the deceased, as well as the medicolegal implication for the clinician performing the procedure, since, theoretically, assault charges could be leveled at the clinician.

The advent of the practice of freezing sperm from adolescent patients[4] has also elicited interest in becoming a grandparent posthumously. Likewise, the freezing of oocytes and ovarian tissue adds new dimensions to posthumous parenting. The potential for cryopreservation of ova may extend the options for posthumous reproduction to the use of cryopreserved oocytes, which would be similar to using sperm for posthumous conception. With advances in cryopreservation technology, more women could consider the possibility of producing a child with their genetic material after death, given that the initial impetus for storing is to protect their own fertility. This process could be carried out, because there are currently no statutes prohibiting posthumous reproduction by women, and surrogacy is allowed. The combination of surrogacy and intracytoplasmic sperm injection (ICSI) make posthumous parenting possible in these very unusual circumstances, which would add considerable social and legal complexity to the status of the child[5]. The probability that these options will be pursued depends on national laws, and the quality of information, the support and the counseling that the bereaved are given.

THE NEED FOR CONSENT

The title of this section suggests that the provider of the sperm also has a choice, and prior informed consent is a crucial basis upon which to proceed to posthumous assisted reproduction (PAR). Around the world, the intention of the deceased has a profound impact on the decision-making process involved in PAR.

Any coherent ethical framework in the area of PAR must be sensitive to the many interests at stake. It is all too easy to overlook the interests of the dead, as the dead have no voice. Some may claim that we cannot speak sensibly of the dead as having interests which can be harmed by the conduct of surviving parties, because, once a person dies, concepts of harm or benefit are redundant. Certain acts committed after a person's death can, however, affect that individual's interests; for example, a posthumous event that destroys a deceased person's reputation harms his or her interests.

Our society has developed procedures that allow us to control certain matters after death, such as the transfer of property, or the transplantation of organs. It is important that individuals have the assurance that their bodies will not be used in a manner inconsistent with their expectations. Even if there is evidence that the deceased desired parenthood in life, it is a considerable leap to assume that he or she would have wished to become a parent posthumously.

If the deceased person's wishes are to be safeguarded adequately, clear evidence of intent to reproduce after death should be required. The potential for a serious conflict of interest justifies a limited decision-making role for the family. Difficulties could arise in estate distribution after PAR, although no cases are yet documented.

Policy-makers must identify and evaluate important interests, and codify them in a workable policy. The UK Human Fertilisation and Embryology (HFE) Act 1990 provides exemplary directions as to the need for written and informed consent prior to any storage and use of gametes or embryos. Contentious areas remain, however, such as the non-recognition of inheritance rights (although the genetic father may now be included on the birth certificate if he has previously consented)[6].

CASES

Numerous cases around the world have been reported whereby sperm have been utilized posthumously. In recent times, Mrs Diane Blood's case has contributed significantly to our understanding of the HFE Act 1990, the nature of informed and written consent, the notion of paternity after posthumous birth of a child and the importance of European Union (EU) law. This landmark UK case involved Mrs Blood[7], whose comatose husband's sperm were retrieved surgically and frozen upon her request, after which the patient died. It was deemed that effective consent, which must be in written form, was not in place before the taking and freezing of gametes. It was even felt that there may have been a case for pressing assault charges against the clinician who undertook the retrieval procedure. The taking of the sperm sample by the clinician was understandable given that the opportunity would otherwise have been lost forever, together with the fact that no guiding case or precedent existed. The importance and strength of the need for written informed consent in relation to the HFE Act 1990 became more apparent to practitioners in the field only after this case, and it made it inevitable that the practice of gaining written informed consent prior to sperm storage was tightened. Had the sperm been retrieved and not frozen but used immediately, however, then the provisions of the HFE Act 1990, s4(1)(b) would not have applied.

In the UK, and to some extent in Europe, an added dimension is the increased power that individual patients possess thanks to the Human Rights Act[8]. This declares that public bodies should not interfere with privacy or family life unless they can justify it in terms of protecting public health or morals, or protecting the rights of others. This additional piece of legislation helped to some extent to gain the right for the deceased father to be named on the birth certificate, when previously the child born posthumously was classified as being 'fatherless'.

Having outlined the legal and ethical issues, the moral question arises of what prompted Mrs Blood to create a child who would be deprived of a living father even before conception. It is evident that she had read about the possibility of this technology in some magazine and the couple had discussed the possibility and that Stephen, her husband, had agreed to this approach. Furthermore, she had spoken to her late husband about having children; she had taken a marriage vow with the purpose of having children; and she felt supported by both sets of parents who could act effectively to promote the welfare of the child as grandparents. Mrs Blood also asserted that she could have used donor sperm or any other person's sperm, but this was quite meaningless for her given the marriage vow taken with Stephen. In the end, although the Appeals Court agreed with the High Court judge in so far as the need for written informed consent, it stated that the Human Fertilisation and Embryology Authority (HFEA) was perhaps overly concerned with setting a precedent, and not properly informed on EU directives. Although the sperm samples were released, they could not be used in the UK, and *in vitro* fertilization (IVF) treatment took place in Belgium.

Mrs Blood always asserted her desire to be away from the media once pregnancy had ensued, but the gravity of the issues involved and public interest meant that her pregnancy and life to follow would be under the microscope in a manner that no other case previously had been. Her subsequent story was elicited by a medical journalist attending a conference in Sweden, which further illustrates the need to guard patient confidentiality in such environments. This case highlights her strong sense of the importance of a marriage vow as expressing an intention to have children. She had clearly thought through the welfare of the child issues and the need for a father or father figure, as stated in the HFE Act 1990, and now she is a proud mother of two boys and well supported by two sets of grandparents and well-wishers.

In a further revealing and unique insight into what happened in the aftermath of posthumous insemination/conception, Mrs Blood describes vivid details. In her own words, 'whenever I dreamt of the baby it was always a boy. I dreamt the night the baby was conceived Steph (Stephen) visited me in my hotel bedroom. I kept asking him questions, but he appeared unable to talk. Instead he took a piece of paper and drew on it. First an "I" and then a heart. I expected him to continue with a "U", but he drew a person. I thought he must be drawing me, but it was a boy'. Following this description, the detail of what went on during delivery is equally striking: 'Liam Stephen was making a funny snoring-type of noise. The midwife explained that he was having difficulty breathing and they were going to take him to the special care unit. She seemed calm but the snoring reminded me of the noise Stephen had made just before his breathing arrested in hospital and he'd suffered a heart attack that heralded his death.' Diane Blood looked helplessly into the incubator with tears running down her cheeks. 'As time progressed Liam was not getting well. The similarities between Stephen's final few days and Liam's first few days, together with the brain scans, wires and tubes attached to the body, were quite distressing. Liam looked a lot like Stephen'[9].

We can all be grateful to Diane Blood for sharing such intimate details with the outside world. The depth of feelings, love, devotion and sense of an ongoing 'relationship' with her late husband are also striking, which would all the more provide a justification for creating a meaningful family for her. On reflection, therefore, there can be little objection to her choice be a parent posthumously. The choice was dictated by her feelings about what was right for her and her family, and did not need moral guidance from outside. The widow was calm and focused, with clear ideas of what she wanted, whilst being well supported. Equally, the UK law did not wish to act as moral guardian in the case, but it was clear and correct in objecting to the use of sperm where no written informed consent pre-existed, a central tenet of the HFE Act 1990.

Whilst this case is unlikely to be repeated in the UK, numerous cases are likely to occur around the world where death is unanticipated and the strict controls that are in place in the UK do not exist. Requests for sperm retrieval are likely to be considered by *ad hoc* ethics committees or by consultants with ethics backgrounds, taking very big decisions about people's lives.

It is with this thought that we turn next to the interest of the deceased, as unreal as it may sound. Posthumous conception redefines the content and outlines of the deceased's life. When it occurs without the person's consent, it deprives an individual of the opportunity to be the author of a highly significant event in his or her life. This is one of the reasons why an analogy between posthumous conception and organ donation fails: procreation is central to an individual's identity in a way that organ donation is not. Respect for autonomy requires that this procedure should not be permitted unless the deceased's consent is clear.

We consider more cases that shed light on the decision-making process which may or may not create the chance to become a parent posthumously. The following two cases were reported the in USA[10]. First, a 28-year-old man, married for 6 years, was childless. After a bout of depression and marital separation for 3 months, he started antidepressant medication. However, 2 weeks later he was brought in by paramedics with a self-inflicted gun wound. He is the only child of his parents, and just before he died they requested the intensive-care physician to arrange for sperm retrieval so that they might have a grandchild with the estranged wife, with whom reconciliation was contemplated, which would enable the genetic line to continue. A clinical ethics consultant reviewed the case and was unable to elicit any substantiating evidence from his widow, and sperm retrieval was denied.

In a second case, a 36-year-old previously healthy man was admitted with pneumonia. After having developed adult respiratory distress syndrome requiring assisted ventilation, 14 days of aggressive treatment followed, leading eventually to multiorgan failure. His wife was informed that he could not survive, and she requested sperm harvest so that she could still have a child. An ethics consultation was requested, and it transpired that they had been trying for a child for 10 years, and 2 months before his death they had seen a fertility specialist and IVF treatment was to begin in the next menstrual cycle. Although there was evidence of his desire to become a father, this alone could not be construed as consent for the collection of sperm for use posthumously. There had been discussion of the nature of single-motherhood and of the welfare of the child. Although she acknowledged that they had never discussed the possibility of posthumous reproduction, the wife believed that he would have wanted this, a presumption supported by his sister. His sister revealed his wish to continue the family line and a strong will to have children. His physicians, nurses and ethics consultant believed that the available information adequately supported his wife's expression of his presumed wishes. Within one hour of his death, his epididymides were removed and frozen. Both cases highlight the constraints of time, available information and personnel involved in the decision-making process. The common theme is genetic perpetuity and the desire to have the deceased's child on the part of a reproductive partner and parents.

Other cases involving posthumous parenting have enriched our knowledge in different ways. The issues arising from a child born through PAR attracted debate in 1983 when Mario and Elsa Rios died in a plane crash, leaving behind two frozen pre-embryos in an IVF clinic in Melbourne, Australia. The question of when life began was considered by the courts in deciding whether the embryos could inherit the couple's $8 million. The Tasmanian judge felt that embryos had the potential to become human beings and therefore could inherit. An independent group set up to look at the case, however, concluded that the embryos would better serve the interests of science; they were donated for research instead of being made available to another infertile couple[11].

In the case of *Hecht* vs. *Superior Court*, the children of William Kane battled with Kane's lover over possession of sperm that Kane deposited in a sperm bank with the express intention that Hecht, his girlfriend, would use the sperm to conceive children after Kane committed suicide. A conflict arose, with opposition to posthumous sperm use by Kane's adult children. The court was faced with the question of whether sperm was something a person could leave to another through a will[12].

Kane, who had been storing sperm, gave his girlfriend 15 vials of semen and then committed suicide. His adult children challenged the gift, arguing that the sperm should be destroyed because there were no property rights attached to sperm. The court did not accept the children's position, arguing that sperm was property for the purposes of devise and for the probate court to have jurisdiction over. The court, however, refused to apply more general property principles. The court also noted the American Fertility Society's position that 'gametes and conceptuses were the property of donors'. In addition, donors have the right to decide at their sole discretion the disposition of these items, provided such disposition is within medical ethical guidelines. The court recognized that sperm and embryos stored solely for the purpose of artificial insemination are 'unlike other human tissue because it is gametic material that can be used for reproduction'. The court reasoned that the value of sperm lies in the potential to create a child after fertilization. Ultimately, the court did not award the sperm to the girlfriend, because the issue before the court was simply whether a lower court properly ordered the sperm to be destroyed. Instead, the court reversed that order, holding that the sperm was entitled to be distributed in probate. Thereafter, the probate court ruled that the girlfriend, based on a distribution formula in a settlement agreement, was entitled to 20% of the frozen semen.

Although the issue of sperm as property is unsettled and complicated, the issue is even more problematic with respect to eggs, primarily because it is rare for unfertilized eggs to be cryopreserved. Nonetheless, the analysis of the Hecht court in finding a limited property right in sperm and finding the value of sperm to be in its potential to create a child could be similarly applied to eggs harvested to be used later for reproduction. Moreover, given the American Fertility Society's position on gametes as donor property, it would be inconsistent for them to view eggs as anything other than property.

The Hecht court was very concerned that gametic material should be used as the donor intended. One way to enable individuals to have their materials used as intended is by recognizing human biological materials as property, thereby giving the owner an enforceable stake in them. One can argue, however, that property rights in human biological materials should be recognized because of the protective value of the rights, and because it will provide a relatively unified approach to settling the complicated issues that arise where the status and disposition of human biological materials are concerned[13]. Yet many people are opposed to recognizing property rights in the human body, arguing that it commodifies the body and demeans human dignity.

Whilst it might seem unusual that a parent of a deceased child would want to create a grandchild from the deceased child's biological materials, it would not be the first time that such a request has been made. For example, Pamela Reno of Reno, Nevada, was devastated when her 19-year-old son killed himself playing Russian roulette. Although her son had wanted to donate his organs in the event of his death, she refused to permit doctors to take them unless they harvested her son's sperm. The doctors collected and cryopreserved his sperm, which she plans to use to impregnate her son's childhood friend and then raise the children – her grandchildren – herself. Reno explained that she desperately wanted grandchildren and that her son always wanted to have children, so she was merely fulfilling his wish by creating his son. While this situation is slightly different from one that could arise with respect to the materials of deceased child-participants, in that the materials have already been collected and preserved, it underscores the fact that previously unimaginable issues can arise in the context of assisted reproductive technologies. Thus, although this scenario is quite bizarre, we must realize that issues such as this could arise if a child who stores gametes then dies, because, as the doctor who harvested Pam Reno's son's sperm stated, this is 'a request that is becoming more frequent'[14].

Posthumous parenting has occurred in potentially infective circumstances, but this risk was already being taken when both partners were alive and IVF treatment was pursued. A human immunodeficiency virus (HIV)-discordant couple failed to conceive through *in vitro* fertilization and ICSI of cryopreserved semen banked by the HIV-positive partner. The husband developed acquired immunodeficiency syndrome (AIDS) and died. A subsequent frozen embryo transfer resulted in pregnancy, and both mother and child were HIV negative[15]. In this case, perhaps more detailed consideration could have been undertaken by both partners and clinical support staff, given that death was a real possibility and preparation for posthumous procreation was a real prospect.

In another slightly controversial case, the Brisbane Supreme Court denied an Australian woman's request to harvest and freeze her dead fiancé's sperm for PAR. After she was denied access to the sperm, the woman learnt that her fiancé may have been a sperm donor, and she began finding out whether his sperm was still available[16]. Given what we know, there is a good ethical argument that the woman should have access to the sperm and be allowed to have her dead fiancé's child. After all, she could use the semen sample if available from the donor sperm perspective.

A few recent cases include those of a husband who drowned in a swimming pool; in a landmark ruling, the Queensland Supreme Court (2004) approved the collection of semen, but use was subject to a further court order. The taking of a sample was influenced by the fact that the couple had lived together for 5 years and had been married for 4 months. The purpose of marriage was to have children. In 2003, a North Queensland woman requested sperm harvest following her fiancé's fall over a waterfall. The partner cited the fact that the couple had taken out holiday insurance together to cover 'family', and that this indication would support their will to have a family. The request to harvest was turned down by the court, as it felt that the necessary changes in the law should be initiated by parliament. In a different case in the USA, there was an interesting judgment following an application for social security support for 2-year-old twins born posthumously from frozen sperm in a case of leukemia, and where the couple had previously been married for 3.5 years. In denying social support the court had effectively indicated that marriage had ended with death, and that consent should also be for child support and not only posthumous reproduction. In the UK, about 30 births through posthumous use of sperm are estimated. In one case, Diane Scott, 44 years of age, after five IVF attempts and 30 months after the death of her husband gave birth to a girl[17]. She acknowledged that it was not ideal to be single parent, but she was supported by friends. Significantly, she said: '*a part of him is ongoing*'.

OUR EXPERIENCE

Our unit stores sperm from men who are about to receive potentially gonadotoxic treatment, and some men may unfortunately die through the nature of the illness. We would not entertain the possibility of sperm harvest without written consent being in place unless the courts or coroner have advised us accordingly. What is clear in the aftermath of death is the bereaved's overwhelming interest in keeping the sperm[18]. In fact there is a desperate need for the surviving partner, widow or parent to check whether frozen sperm are still in place, and to be assured that they will not be discarded without their permission. The common thread which runs though the numerous cases is that the frozen semen sample signifies to them that the deceased or part of him is still alive, and reassurance is gained that these samples will not be discarded. However, in the UK, the sperm can only be kept frozen and used in line with the wishes of the deceased. The next element that follows is counseling with a therapeutic and supportive role, whereby the surviving may talk about the deceased and describe their lives when alive. Without fail they tell you of what reassurance and comfort it is for them to know that frozen sperm is still in place and how they wish it to remain in storage for the foreseeable future. As time progresses it becomes clear that the use of sperm seems a distant objective. The eventual decision to discard it occurs when a new and stable man enters their life, or they realise that they have crossed the threshold to have a child naturally. The other circumstance is when the partner fully accepts the deceased's death. There have been specific instances where friction between the surviving partner and the deceased's family members has occurred, and where tension has centered on issues of inheritance and the sharing of an estate. Parents are increasingly seeking ways to keep the frozen sperm with a view to grandparenting, keeping the family name alive, hiring a surrogate and replacing the deceased. Practically all the complex issues have been dealt with by means of careful and sensitive dialog, consultation and counseling, with a view to upholding the will and autonomy of the deceased. This has been the advantage of written informed consent being in place. Successful dialog and counseling has also meant that those seeking posthumous reproduction have accepted fully the reality of the process without being under duress, and this may have come about by facilitating access to other team members such as the consultant and an independent counselor. Whilst expressions of a serious intention to proceed have occurred, none has so far materialized into action. Throughout, we have adopted a neutral position in relation to the posthumous use of sperm.

In our clinic, among requests by 21 new widows to keep frozen sperm, there has been little evidence of its subsequent use, which reflects just how strong the psychological bond was with the deceased, and the complex process of mourning that ensues[18]. After 7 years, even those 11 widows who stated their intention to use frozen sperm did not resort to PAR. Their desire to continue to maintain the sperm without use is another important aspect of the grieving process. We are aware of two widows who, once in a newly found, stable relationship, requested disposal of the deceased's sperm sample. It is therefore important to formulate a mourning period of 1–1.5 years when no insemination should occur, during which counseling should be provided.

With one of the largest adolescent cancer patients' storage facilities in the UK we have had several patients in this category who have since died, and five parents and one grandparent who have come forward to express an interest in creating a grandchild and great-grandchild. Whilst support and therapeutic counseling and consultation was conducted, each was told of the clear-cut position in the UK of the need to have a named partner with whom treatment could occur, which was impossible given that they were young and single. The use of a surrogate was routinely raised, and apart from the information we could provide, each bereaved person was routinely asked to seek independent legal advice or seek information from the HFEA directly. The HFEA, apart from its regulatory function, also helps to support public and patient welfare. Two cases in the past 20 years involving adult patients centered on a significant conflict of interest over an inheritance between the family of the deceased and the bereaved reproductive partner, which would be affected by the procreation of a child posthumously.

Eventually, disposal of the sperm sample is chosen, and one widow's exemplary response to us was:

> *You are probably aware that the samples were deposited because my husband was about to undergo treatment for cancer that might have left him infertile. Unfortunately, I have to inform you that the treatment was unsuccessful and my husband died. I am sorry that I have not informed you sooner, but to actively write and agree to the disposal of samples was something that I have not been able to do until now. Although in the end I have decided not to make use of the samples, I would like you to know what a comfort it has been, knowing that they were there and the option to have another child was available to me. Had my husband lived I know we would have wanted more children. However, our son was only 15 weeks old when my husband died and at that time I should have had another. I was either still grieving or still optimistic that I would meet someone else and have a baby naturally. Now, I have given up hope having decided I am too old to have another child and that the gap between my son and a new baby would be too great. I am therefore content that the samples be destroyed.*

LEGAL AND SOCIAL STATUS OF THE CHILD

The effects on a child of being the product of posthumous reproduction are not completely understood. Little is known about the psychological effects on a child who eventually learns that one or both parents were dead long before that child's own gestation began. Some experts complain that, in the modern conception industry, the rights and privileges of potential parents have precedence over the welfare of children.

The concern with PAR is that bringing the child into a single-parent household would be harmful to the child. However, a serious problem with this objection is that the act that supposedly harms the child is the very process that brings it into being[19-21]. Persons are harmed only if they are caused to be worse off than they otherwise would have been[22].

If pregnancy and birth occur within the context of marriage in which one partner has died, the effects on the child might not be very different to those which occur in the much more common case of posthumous birth, in terms of legitimacy and inheritance. The psychological impact on the child should be minimal, and probably within the range of experiences seen in some parallel studies on, for example, single-parent families[23,24].

Some states in the USA have adopted the Uniform Parentage Act, according to which the deceased man would be presumed to be the father of the child provided that the couple had been married and the birth occurred within 300 days of the man's death[25]. If birth occurs after 300 days in those states, or if birth occurs in states without statutes addressing posthumous conception, then current law provides no basis for presuming that the deceased is the legal father[25].

In considering the welfare of the child, the Takamatsu High Court (2004) in Japan recognized parental responsibility and objective evidence of a blood relationship, and gave high priority to the legitimacy of family lineage. Equally there was fear of endorsing posthumous reproduction. In contrast, the Matsuyama District Court (2003) in Japan earlier had not recognized the legitimacy of the offspring born through posthumous means, but did recognize the child's welfare and dignity and that a degree of understanding was needed, given that the laws were inadequate. In 2005, Japan was to see new legislation which may clarify, for instance, inheritance and right of ownership of sperm, but the New Bill appears to avoid the mention of posthumous reproduction. In 2004, the Sacramento Assembly, USA, recognized that children born in posthumous circumstances will have inheritance rights. The UK situation has also changed: no longer is a child considered fatherless in cases of posthumous insemination; now a father is recognized on the birth certificate, if the father in life had consented to this when living[6]. However, inheritance rights in the UK do not follow from this recognition, a somewhat obtuse position given the increasing emphasis on considering the welfare of the child.

THE FUTURE

Decisions concerning whether or not to have a child have been considered a private matter and a fundamental human right, but there are limited precedents regarding how this might be respected after one's death. In the UK, it is imperative that the donor has given written, informed consent, and it is illegal to store sperm, oocytes or embryos without the written consent of the genetic provider(s) under the HFE Act 1990[26]. Furthermore, in the UK, and to some extent Europe, there are added dimensions about the increased power that individual patients possess thanks to the Human Rights Act[8]. This declares that public bodies should not interfere with privacy or family life unless they can justify it in terms of protecting public health or morals, or protecting the rights of others. It means that the decision whether or not to become a parent does not justify intervention by public bodies in the main, and decisions are necessarily individual and should be made on a case by case basis.

Most people do not expect that their gametes will be used for procreation after death, so generally do not make their views regarding this practice explicit. However, it is both unfair and undesirable to place the onus upon individuals to state their opposition to posthumous conception. From our experience it is clearer that, given more time and support, the widow or surviving partner is unlikely to proceed with posthumous insemination. Whether there is opposition through the hospital, establishment or authorities remains as yet an undetermined but probable contributing factor in the decision actively to use the sperm. Our work shows also that more time and attention need to be given to supporting those surviving partners. It raises the question as to what should be the time interval, or period in which no insemination should occur, as decisions made immediately after the partner's death are more likely to be based on emotion. Perhaps a 12–18-month grace period would help the widow to reach a more rational decision. The position and attitude of clinics will also have a profound effect on the motivation of the widow. It may be inconsistent for a public body, and contrary to the Human Rights Act 1998, to adopt a blanket ban policy[8]. Individual members of clinics, laboratory and other staff members, who object to posthumous reproduction may withdraw from assisting with the process through the clause of conscientious objection laid in the HFE Act 1990. There is a call for protocols to be developed for posthumous reproduction[27,28].

Future developments in the field of *in vitro* maturation of gametes have recognized the potential for using fetal ovaries as an unlimited source of oocytes. The ethical, social and legal issues would be profound if such oocytes were used, since the donor would never have given consent. The psychological well-being of children born to an unborn genetic mother could be profoundly affected by such a situation. Society as a whole would need to face up to the bizarre possibility of a genetic mother, the donor, who had never been born.

WHAT HAVE WE LEARNT SO FAR?

Posthumous reproductive choice exists and may be exercised around the world. Ideally, informed written consent would simplify one aspect, namely the wishes of the dead. Even if frozen sperm are allowed to be used posthumously, there are strong indications that surviving partners are not choosing this option, but take comfort in knowing that the sperm exist for their use. Strong support and therapeutic counseling, and general support for survivors, should be made available. It would be incorrect to obstruct a widow in her self-determination, and indeed, for most hospitals, who in this case function as the public body, such obstruction is contrary to the Human Rights Act 1998[8]; but there is considerable scope for those treating, who object, to withdraw from treatment, at least in the UK. There seems little evidence to suggest that children born through posthumous reproduction could be harmed, although around the world greater effort is needed to secure their welfare and especially inheritance rights. Issues of posthumous reproduction have challenged and enriched our understanding of laws, and our understanding of, for example, the property status of gametes and the status of the child.

Many widows and prospective partners have displayed a special relationship and bond, and shown that marriage or the intention behind marrying was to have children. Marriage took on a special dimension in death to the bereaved, although in one case relating to social security, marriage was deemed to have ended with death. Marriage vows talk of 'till death do us part', but in reality the care of that special relationship and remembrance continues long afterwards. The bereaved strongly express their remembrance of their partner, and the belief that a part of the dead is still ongoing and alive gives comfort to the surviving partner, and a strong reason to face up to new realities. The author sees no harm in this, since the alternative could be severe bouts of depression; advances in reproductive technologies may to some degree contribute in therapeutic ways to the mourning process.

CONCLUSIONS

To be or not to be a parent after one's death will always remain a moot and difficult choice, with several complex facets to it. However, one must not obstruct anyone in their self-determination provided that one is satisfied that the deceased partner may have wanted this, and, although written, informed consent would be highly desirable, cases around the world will occur where presumed wishes will need to be deciphered. The exact reasoning for widows to choose posthumous reproduction remains elusive, but they are generally motivated by strong expressions of love, a desire for remembrance and to make a meaningful choice of genetic partner with whom to have children. After all, donor insemination is widely utilized. Continued support for the bereaved must be in place, especially where services store gametes and embryos from patients suffering from illness. Protocols for posthumous reproduction need to be developed and improved. Cases reported so far show a strong-willed individual choosing posthumous reproduction to apparently satisfy their needs as a parent. The decision to conceive a child posthumously is necessarily driven by the surviving partner, but should also involve adequate counseling and attention to the welfare of the child. The welfare of unborn children needs to be taken into account in a balanced, pragmatic and sensible manner, and especially so that they are not disadvantaged in areas such as inheritance.

REFERENCES

1. Aziza-Shuster E. A child at all costs: posthumous reproduction and the meaning of parenthood. Hum Reprod 1994; 9: 2182–5.
2. Bahadur G. Death and conception. Hum Reprod 2002; 17: 2769–75.

3. Strong C, Gingrich JR, Kutteh WH. Ethics of sperm retrieval after death or persistent vegetative state. Hum Reprod 2000; 15: 739–45.

4. Bahadur G. Semen quality and cryopreservation in adolescent cancer patients. Hum Reprod 2002; 17: 3175–61.

5. Fraser L. Our son is dead, but his sperm survives and we must give him the baby he wanted so much. Mail on Sunday, 19 December 1999.

6. Human Fertilisation and Embryology (Deceased Fathers) Act 2003. London: HMSO, 2003.

7. R vs. Human Fertilisation and Embryology Authority, exp Blood, 1997. 2 All ER 687, (1997) 35 BMLR 1, CA.

8. Bahadur G. The Human Rights Act (1998) and its impact on human reproductive issues. Hum Reprod 2001; 16: 785–9.

9. Blood, D. Flesh and Blood. Edinburgh: Mainstream Press, 2004.

10. Orr RD, Siegler M. Is posthumous semen retrieval ethically permissible? J Med Ethics 2002; 28: 299–303.

11. Smith GP, III. Australia's frozen 'orphan' embryos: a medical, legal, and ethical dilemma. J Family Law 1985–86; 24: 27–41.

12. Hecht vs. Superior Court, 16 Cal.App.4th 836, 20 Cal. Rptr.2d 275 (June 1993).

13. Bahadur G. Ethics of testicular stem cell medicine. Hum Reprod 2004; 19: 2702–10.

14. Anonymous. Now I've got my son's sperm, nothing will stop me becoming a gran. Daily Express, 20 September 2000.

15. Sauer MV, Chang PL. Posthumous reproduction in a human immunodeficiency virus discordant couple. Am J Obstet Gynecol 2001; 185: 252–3.

16. Spriggs M. Woman wants dead fiance's baby: who owns a dead man's sperm. J Med Ethics 2004; 30: 384–8.

17. Laurance J. Baby born 30 months after father's death. The Independent, 4 October 2004.

18. Bahadur G. Posthumous assisted reproduction (PAR) – potential cases, counselling and consent. Hum Reprod 1996; 11: 2573–5.

19. Robertson JA. Children of Choice: Freedom and the New Reproductive Technologies. Princeton, NJ: Princeton University Press, 1994.

20. Robertson JA. Posthumous reproduction. In Kempers RD, Cohen J, Haney AF, et al., eds. Fertility and Reproductive Medicine. New York: Elsevier Science, 1998: 255–9.

21. Strong C. Ethics in Reproductive and Perinatal Medicine: A New Framework. New Haven, CT: Yale University Press, 1997.

22. Feinberg J. Harm to Others. New York: Oxford University Press, 1984.

23. Golombok S. New families, old values: considerations regarding the welfare of the child. Hum Reprod 1998; 13: 2342–7.

24. Pennings G. Measuring the welfare of the child: in search of the appropriate evaluation principle. Hum Reprod 1999; 14: 1146–50.

25. Gibbons JA. Who's your daddy?: a constitutional analysis of post-mortem insemination. J Contemp Health Law Policy 1997; 14: 187–210.

26. Human Fertilisation and Embryology Act 1990. London: HMSO, 1990.

27. Bahadur G. Protocols for posthumous fatherhood. Fertil Steril 2004; 81: 223–4.

28. Batzer F, Hurwitz JM, Caplan A. Posthumous parenthood and the need for a protocol with posthumous sperm procurement. Fertil Steril 2003; 79: 1263–9.

Chapter 4

International parenthood
via procreative tourism

Guido Pennings

Reproductive tourism indicates movements by candidate service recipients from one institution, jurisdiction or country where treatment is not available for them to another institution, jurisdiction or country where they can obtain the kind of medical assistance they desire. Historically, the first movements motivated by the desire to control one's reproduction were for abortions. Even now, yearly, thousands of non-resident women are having an abortion in The Netherlands[1]. The new trend, however, is not about the prevention of conception and/or birth but access to new techniques for infertility treatment. The trend first came to light because of the large media attention for the more extreme cases: a 59-year-old British woman going to Italy to become pregnant, a 62-year-old French woman who went to the United States to be inseminated with her brother's sperm, a British woman who crossed the Channel to Belgium to have a child from her deceased husband, a British couple moving to Spain to select the sex of their future child, etc. There is an almost endless list of more or less unusual applications. Still, when numbers are included in the picture, one realizes that the overwhelming majority of instances of reproductive traveling have little to do with exceptional or strange requests but can be explained by long waiting-lists, lower costs or treatments such as oocyte donation and *in vitro* fertilization (IVF) with donor gametes[2].

SEMANTICS

Concepts and definitions play a crucial role in discussions and arguments. 'Medical tourism', of which 'reproductive tourism' is a part, was originally used for people who went on vacation to exotic places and took advantage of the opportunity to obtain some medical service. Tourism was their primary motive for traveling. This has changed in recent years. The main motive for traveling today is the medical treatment. The exotic and recreational aspect is thrown in as a nice extra. The term 'tourism' clearly has negative connotations when used within a medical context. Tourism refers to traveling for pleasure and out of curiosity. Indirectly, the term devalues the desire motivating the journey: it suggests that the fertility tourist goes abroad to look for something strange and/or trivial. This becomes clear when media reports are analyzed. The term most frequently pops up when applications are presented which are generally condemned as wrong or bizarre. The term 'tourism' expresses the negative evaluation of the cases.

One recent proposal to replace the term 'tourism' is 'reproductive exile'[3]. However, the metaphor used in this alternative is vague. Are the persons banished for something they did or wanted, or are they leaving the country voluntarily because they disagree with the governing rules? Is society or the individual to be blamed for the exile? Whatever the interpretation, the term is never neutral. I propose to replace the term 'reproductive tourism' by 'cross-border reproductive care'. This term has several advantages: it avoids the derogatory meaning of 'tourism', it is objective since it expresses no value judgments regarding traveling, and it fits in with the general term 'cross-border health care' that is commonly used when movements for other health-care services are discussed. It is striking that the term 'tourism' is never mentioned in the parallel discussion that is going on within European circles about 'patient mobility' or 'cross-border health care'. When patient mobility in health care outside the field of reproduction is considered, the general attitude is based on the right of the patient to high-quality health care. The Commission of the European Communities[4] proposes to simplify the existing rules on the coordination of social security systems and the procedures of European health insurance to facilitate patient mobility. Contrary to the attitude towards reproductive care, cross-border movements are positively evaluated as a means to use spare capacity and foreign expertise for the good of the patient. One realizes the extent to which one's views have been molded by the discussion in recent years when one considers what this attitude would mean in the field of reproduction. Countries would be encouraged to inform patients about the possibilities in other countries, patients would receive reimbursement for egg donation abroad if an insufficient number of oocytes is available in one's home country, and so on.

The reason why all this is not happening seems to lie in the fact that the treatment (or a part thereof) offered abroad is legally prohibited in the home country. The negative evaluation of reproductive tourism is triggered by the idea of law evasion. However, if this is the reason, then the condemnation is much too broad. More and more people are traveling, for reasons which have nothing to do with law evasion. Moreover, it is far from clear whether law evasion in this specific context should be ethically condemned.

OTHER SOLUTIONS

The main focus in cross-border reproductive health care is on patient mobility. However, this is only one way to obtain the treatment one desires. All kinds of creative solutions can be imagined. Recently, one website (ManNotIncluded) proposed to send sperm from countries where anonymity is maintained to patients in the United Kingdom. The sample would be delivered with insemination kits directly to a woman's home. Since it would be in a thawing state, the service would (at least according to the organizers) fall outside the remit of the Human Fertilisation and Embryology Authority[5]. Others are thinking of an 'insemination boat', similar to the 'abortion ship' of a Dutch women's organization. Transport of genetic material could also provide a solution. Transport preimplantation genetic diagnosis (PGD) and transport IVF are performed between countries. Some clinics in the United States have a branch in other countries such as Romania, where they collect the eggs and fertilize them with the husband's or partner's sperm, after which the embryos are shipped back to recipients in the United States. The same procedure is applied between clinics in Finland and Russia. In 2003, a Belgian physician caused a major row and a change of law by sending sperm samples to the United States for sperm sorting, to be used later for sex selection for social reasons. Finally, instead of transporting gametes or embryos, one can pay oocyte donors to fly in[6]. Normally, these donations should set off an alarm, since a foreign anonymous donor is a strong indication of payment. However, clinics are not always very strict: the fact that the relationship between donor and recipient is flimsy (or non-existent) does not automatically lead to rejection of the donor. The transportation of donors instead of gametes is more expensive, but it avoids problems such as the language barrier, safety standards, insurance, etc. connected to having treatment in foreign clinics.

CAUSES OF CROSS-BORDER REPRODUCTIVE CARE

It is not easy to study the flows of patients going from one country to another. There exists no monitoring system to track these movements. Moreover, cross-border reproductive care is a multifaceted phenomenon. The general picture has to be composed from diverse and partial snapshots. The main causes of cross-border reproductive care can be summarized as follows:

(1) A type of treatment is forbidden by law because the application is considered ethically unacceptable. For some countries such as Italy, almost every act of medical assistance would fall under this header. One application that is prohibited in most European countries is elective sex selection. People who want to choose whether to have a boy or a girl have to go to the United States or to countries such as Jordan where this desire is accepted[7].

(2) A technique is not available because of lack of expertise or equipment. PGD is a good example. Even in countries where PGD is allowed, not every clinic has the expertise to perform diagnostic tests for all diseases. There may

also be a combination of reasons: technical unavailability may be combined and/or caused by legal restrictions. In one center in Belgium, half of the couples asking for PGD come from Germany and France as a result of legal and practical restrictions in these countries[8].

(3) A treatment is not considered safe enough. This is a complex discussion. Risk is primarily an ethical and not a technical issue. Risk is calculated by multiplying the degree of harm by the probability of this harm. However, even if we were able to measure risk (not an easy task given the difficulty of objective quantification of harm), we still need a moral standard to decide whether the risk is acceptable or not[9]. Especially in the starting phase of a new technique or new variant of an old technique, such as intracytoplasmic sperm injection (ICSI) with non-ejaculated sperm, the use of frozen oocytes or ooplasm transfer, the views on what is acceptable may differ. Even for standard practices, there may be disagreement about acceptable risk. The discussion on the number of embryos to transfer to balance success and multiple pregnancies illustrates this nicely. Most European countries adopt a different standard from the United States where the replacement of three embryos is not considered a problem.

(4) Certain categories of patients are not eligible for assisted reproduction. These are mainly groups such as lesbians or single women, who do not fit into the 'ideal family' of the stable heterosexual couple. Another major group excluded by a normative idea on normal reproduction and parenthood is that of postmenopausal women. In a number of countries, including France, only women of reproductive age have access to infertility treatment.

(5) The waiting-lists are too long in the home country. In some states, there are waiting-lists for standard IVF. In almost all countries in which neither payment nor anonymity is accepted for donors, the shortage of donor gametes is the main cause of long waiting-lists. This applies especially to donor oocytes, but recently also to donor sperm. Both are scarce resources for which people are prepared to travel. This may be due to a combination of factors. People may leave the country because there is a shortage of donors due to the abolition of donor anonymity and simultaneously because they do not want an identifiable donor.

(6) The costs to be paid by patients are too high in their home country.

Revealing the main causes of infertility traveling is important, since the present reaction by policy makers is solely focused on those cases that are motivated by the wish to avoid restrictive legislation. However, precisely for such cases, cross-border traveling should be seen as a safety valve which prevents moral conflict in a democracy, rather than as a threat (see below, 'Tolerance in a pluralistic society').

JUSTICE

The classic argument against reproductive tourism is the inequality of access. Only people with the necessary financial means can afford to look for treatment abroad. Although this is largely correct, this argument entails much more than those who present it might like. If discrimination on the basis of financial means is the prime concern for those who condemn cross-border reproductive care, it follows that their first efforts should be directed at the current reimbursement system. Most countries do not reimburse all costs for all IVF cycles, and a large part of infertility treatment is performed in profit-based private hospitals. In countries where health insurance is largely privatized, most insurance companies do not cover infertility treatment. As a consequence, almost all countries discriminate against patients on the basis of income even for those interventions that are accepted in their country. Those who use the justice argument should first eliminate the existing financial discrimination by guaranteeing public funding of infertility treatment or obligatory insurance coverage. Ironically, when lower financial cost is the reason for crossing the border, injustice is reduced by the possibility of cross-border care, since poor people from rich countries can now obtain treatment they could never afford at home.

A final thought occurs about this financial selection. Most people will agree that universal legal prohibition of certain applications is highly unlikely. The one possible exception, i.e. reproductive cloning, has been blocked very efficiently by the opponents of therapeutic cloning. If universal agreement cannot be reached, one should try to reach uniformity within continents or another, smaller, unit. This goal, however, increases discrimination on the basis of income; it is more expensive for a European citizen to fly to the United States or India to have some treatment than to fly to a neighboring country.

There is another argument hidden beneath the previous one. Some people blame reproductive travelers for using the escape route; they should suffer like the others who do not have the money to travel. 'This raises the question of whether it is equitable, within the EU, that Member States may impose their regulatory choices only on those who cannot afford to "choose" another regulatory regime, by buying a service in another Member State, or to put it the other way, whether it is equitable that some people can in effect "buy their way out" of ethical or moral choices given legislative force in their own Member State'[10]. Reproductive tourists are seen as disloyal, as 'circumventing national laws'[11], as 'evading their domestic constraints'[12], as 'health care shopping . . . where the law may be more lax'[13]. The first question is whether the state is justified in imposing a moral view on citizens who do not consent to these rules and principles. In addition, is it equitable when a state denies its citizens access to a reproductive service that is considered perfectly acceptable in another member state? Finally, as Engelhardt argued a long time ago, envy is a very bad advisor in matters of distributive justice in health care[14].

MORAL TRUTH AND LEGAL UNIFORMITY

Den Hartogh[15] argued that the basic drive for wanting uniformity of legal regulations is a commitment to moral truth. If you are convinced that cloning is wrong, then you should try to prevent people from cloning regardless of where they are. The discussion in the United Nations illustrates this position. The call to ban certain applications of assisted reproductive technology and other forms of research on a worldwide scale is growing louder as politicians are increasingly aware of the possibility of scientists and patients being able to move abroad to circumvent legislation. The attempt to ban human cloning, including research cloning, currently put before the United Nations (UN) illustrates this trend. This move, however, goes in the wrong direction. Instead of trying to prevent others from doing what one thinks is wrong by laws and regulations, one should engage in a moral debate based on persuasion and rational arguments. It is rather difficult to have an open debate when one has absolute confidence about one's own position, as is shown by the opponents in the strong wording that they use: cloning 'is morally repugnant, unethical and contrary to respect for the person'. The analogy between embryonic stem cell research and terrorism made in the UN proposal of Costa Rica demonstrates the same spirit[16]. The analogy clearly shows the commitment to moral truth. However, even regarding terrorism there is disagreement as to who is a terrorist and who a freedom fighter.

The belief in a universal moral truth is also expressed in the reaction of Human Genetics Alert[17] to the Select Committee on Science and Technology of the UK Parliament: 'There is precedent in other legislation for people to be convicted in the UK for acts committed abroad which are legal but illegal in Britain. It should also be made an offence for reproductive technology practitioners to refer people to clinics abroad for the use of technologies illegal in the UK. The Government should make the utmost effort towards promotion of the international harmonisation of legislation and the discouragement of reproductive tourism'. At no point do the authors of this document seem to have considered the possibility that legal harmonisation may force the UK to change its laws. Germany has adopted this view in the context of embryo research. German researchers who collaborate with international colleagues to create new embryonic stem-cell lines are acting illegally[18]. If this attitude is transferred to the field of reproduction, this would imply that every patient and physician who commits acts abroad which are illegal in his or her home country is liable to prosecution when returning. This is one of the most coercive and repressive manners of preventing cross-border reproductive care. Germany has built itself a reputation with this approach. Already in 1990, German border guards forced gynecological examinations upon women coming back from The Netherlands in search of evidence of extraterritorial abortions[19]. Prosecutors also brought criminal charges against women who obtained abortions in other countries.

DANGERS

Although cross-border reproductive care offers several considerable benefits, its dangers should not be underestimated or ignored. A number of these dangers are mere speculations about possible negative side-effects of these movements. It has, for instance, been argued that the influx of patients will increase prices and thus make infertility treatment inaccessible for local couples. Other dangers are slowly but surely corroborated by evidence.

One danger of traveling is that the rights of patients are not respected. Recently, several cases of misconduct on the part of physicians came to light. Two cases presented at a meeting at the European Parliament by the lawyer of the victims revealed serious shortcomings in the way that things are handled in some Romanian clinics[20]. Lack of informed consent, no information about possible health risks and no follow-up of oocyte donors are amongst these points. However, these cases are different in one important respect from most other instances of cross-border reproductive care. The infractions mentioned above are violations of Romanian law and could happen because of a lack of control and supervision. Most services for which people travel are fully within the law of the servicing country.

The issues of informed consent and good clinical practice should be separated from the payment question, although violation of regulations or a lax application of the rules is to a certain extent connected to commercialization. Research conducted in the United States showed, for instance, that the information about risks and complications provided to candidate oocyte donors was not objective and complete[21]. Payment holds the danger of exploitation of women, especially in countries with a high number of very poor people.

Another danger concerns the lack of counseling because of insufficient knowledge of a common language. This problem has already drawn attention from psychologists in the field of assisted reproduction because of the difficulties experienced when counseling immigrants. One possible solution is to provide translators, but most counselors are not happy with this kind of 'indirect' counseling. Another possibility is that the local clinic, most often the clinic where the patients receive their initial treatment or diagnosis, offers counseling before patients leave for treatment abroad. If patient welfare is a primary concern, this option deserves serious consideration. However, this raises the tricky question of complicity when people desire a treatment that is legally prohibited in the home country. Still, it is a real option in certain countries. In Switzerland, no specific addresses of service providers abroad may be given to patients, neither may collaboration with foreign centers be established, but it is allowed to provide counseling for oocyte donation although this treatment is forbidden in Switzerland[22]. However, lack of counseling may not only be caused by language difficulties. For-profit clinics may have a strong tendency to focus on the technical–medical aspect of the intervention and ignore the psychosocial side of infertility treatment.

The most important danger concerns control of quality and safety standards. Quality is primarily measured as the take-home baby rate, but numerous other standards have been proposed in the literature. The main result of this discussion is that numbers are difficult to interpret for patients. An international consensus on two or three standards would be welcome. All clinics could then present their results in terms of these standards. However, given the commercial context in which infertility clinics are situated, results inevitably function as publicity. The 'league tables' in the United Kingdom have made this clear. The clinic profits from boosting its results since it will attract more patients. Without careful and thorough control by an independent organization, the numbers must be taken at face value. A regulatory body to monitor success rates and other relevant information (such as complication and multiple pregnancy rates) is essential to guarantee correct patient information. Apparently, Global Egg Donation Resource[23] has something similar in mind: to provide accurate information for those seeking egg donation. Perhaps the most important measure to prevent patients from being lured into low-cost clinics is education about general rules to evaluate certain information, such as the need to take into account the multiple pregnancy rate when comparing the success rate of clinics.

Safety refers to standards for donor screening for transmittable diseases (both genetic and non-genetic), complication rates, multiple pregnancies, morbidity due to ovarian hyperstimulation, etc. Some have argued that a legal framework should solely focus on licensing and controlling centers of assisted reproduction, with the aim of ensuring homogeneous and adequate standards[24]. Patients all over the world have the right to be protected against incompetence, negligence and recklessness on the part of practitioners. Control and legislation should be distinguished: some countries may have good rules and laws but the rules and laws are not checked and enforced, while other countries may just lack enforceable rules. The results for patients will probably be the same. There are indications that some doctors are moving to specific countries precisely to avoid regulations designed to protect patients[20]. The same motive may underlie shifting experiments or risky techniques (such as nuclear transfer) to countries where regulations are less protective of human research subjects[25].

One way to solve this problem is by setting up a system to accredit clinics worldwide so that every patient can be sure that these clinics, wherever they are, operate according to the rules of good clinical practice. In the 1960s, the Association to Repeal Abortion Laws (ARAL) provided American women with a list of physicians in Mexico and Japan who performed abortions. This association simultaneously created mechanisms in order to ensure the quality of the abortionists, thus giving them a 'license'[26]. In fact, this evolution may be stimulated not so much by concerns for the welfare of patients but by basic economic rules; if accredited clinics attract more patients than non-accredited clinics, they have a financial incentive to obtain accreditation. A last argument for promoting such a system from the aspect of the home countries of travelers is again financial, as it is generally the home country which bears the costs of complications. When people take risks going abroad to cheaper but unsafe clinics, the final payer might be the health insurance of their home country. When three or more embryos are replaced, this may increase the success rate of the providing clinic while the medical costs of higher-order multiple pregnancies are shipped back home. Finally, when things go wrong, the patients have little recourse to local courts. Moreover, malpractice laws may not even exist in some of these countries.

A MARKET OF REPRODUCTIVE SERVICES

Within the European context, health care is more and more considered as a product or service like any other. The European Court of Justice ruling in Decker and Kohll has made mainstream health services subject to two principles on which the European Union was founded: the freedom of movement of goods and the freedom of movement of services. Health care is now deemed to be tradable[27]. The right to free movement is an intrinsic part of the conception of European citizenship as a 'market citizenship'. This concept refers to the individualistic variant of liberalism and presents citizenship as a set of entitlements to facilitate market integration. 'Such an approach draws on the liberal conception of citizenship as a status bestowed on morally autonomous individuals who pursue their chosen forms of life'[28]. Contrary to the first impression one gets when listening to the reactions on reproductive cross-border care, these movements fit nicely into the main framework of the European Union.

The increasing commercialization of health care can be noticed on several points. Hospitals are spending a lot of money on publicity to attract wealthy patients from other countries. A number of countries, especially Asian states such as India and Thailand, are counting on this revenue as an important part of their gross domestic product. Health care abroad has become a multibillion dollar industry. To make things easier for patients, clinics offer package deals that include flights, visas, hotels, personal assistants and translators. The clinics are also explicitly pointing out price differences compared with other countries for the same surgical intervention or treatment. The general marketing strategies do not differ from those used for selling cars or any other product.

TOLERANCE IN A PLURALISTIC SOCIETY

The majority in a democracy has the right to impose rules that correspond with their view on 'the good life' and their view on how society should be organized. Indeed, this is what politics is all about. Political parties try to put their moral stamp on societal institutions such as the law. The present law in Italy on assisted reproduction illustrates this nicely[29]. This law is clearly based on a single moral position, i.e. the Catholic religion. The majority of Italian members of parliament, as representatives of those who elected them, voted in favor of this law.

As a democrat, it is difficult to find any fault in this procedure. Still, opponents to the law managed to assemble four million signatures to hold a referendum to change the law. This is a very strong signal to the majority in parliament that a large part of the population rejects the regulation. The question now becomes why Italians who disagree with this law should not look for treatment abroad.

Although the majority has the political right to impose its view, this right should be balanced against ethical values and principles. Among these values, we count tolerance, autonomy and respect for others' opinion. One conclusion which follows from these values is that governments should not use their repressive power to control the behavior of their citizens in personal matters. The possibility of citizens circumventing the legislation by going abroad demands a specific view on the function of the law. Legislation can still function as a public statement on the moral convictions of the majority, but legislation can no longer assure that the citizens of a country will not make use of certain medical services. This already influences the way lawmakers evaluate new law proposals. The Swiss Federal Council argued against a referendum initiative that intended to prohibit most forms of IVF and the use of donor gametes because the only consequence of such law would be the flight of infertile couples to neighboring countries[30]. Obviously, this argument did not convince the Italian lawmakers. Eventually, accepting this fact may lead to a more liberal law by taking into account the desires and convictions of minority groups in society. If one wishes to prevent cross-border reproductive care and law evasion, one should not introduce its major cause, i.e. restrictive legislation. Moreover, the fact that one European member state (sharing the same great culture and values, if Europhiles are to be believed) allows and finds perfectly legitimate a treatment that another member state wants to prohibit at all costs should raise a flicker of doubt in the minds of both. This doubt should result in a minimal form of tolerance towards citizens with a different view (in their home country) by allowing them to obtain the treatment they desire abroad. Allowing one's citizens cross-border reproductive care demonstrates the absolute minimum of respect for their moral autonomy. Preventing by all means minority members from obtaining the treatment they desire would also be dangerous as it would increase feelings of frustration, suppression and indignation. Reproductive traveling should be seen as a safety valve that avoids moral conflict and thus contributes to a peaceful coexistence of different ethical and religious views. Cross-border reproductive care motivated by the wish to avoid legislation that is based on moral convictions not shared by some should not be considered as a problem, but rather should be seen as the solution to an inevitable conflict between politics and ethics in a democracy.

Tolerance is the key issue. This attitude may be the only practical way to handle the diversity of moral opinions that is a basic fact of modern societies. Real tolerance fulfills three conditions: A disapproves of the conduct of B; A has the power to stop or punish B; and A, nevertheless, does not stop or punish the conduct of B but chooses to allow it[31]. The difficult task for A is to explain why he or she allows someone else to do things he or she finds morally repulsive or at least morally wrong when he or she has the possibility to stop it. The Dutch solution, called 'pragmatic tolerance' ('gedogen'), is a policy whereby some acts are legally prohibited but which simultaneously specifies the conditions under which the law-breaker will not be prosecuted. Euthanasia, for instance, is still forbidden by law in The Netherlands but physicians who perform euthanasia will not be prosecuted if certain conditions have been fulfilled. Leaving the territory to obtain a treatment that one is not legally allowed to have at home may be such a condition. On the other hand, cross-border reproductive care may not stem from a form of real tolerance. If people do not broadcast the reason why they leave the country, the state will never know what they plan to do, and consequently does not have the power to stop or punish these citizens.

CROSS-BORDER CARE AS CIVIL DISOBEDIENCE

Instead of looking at cross-border traveling as attempts at law evasion, some instances can be seen as a form of civil disobedience. It is a way of prodding the majority into reconsidering the decision it has taken[32]. The minority demonstrates the intensity of its feelings by disobeying the law. If the law forbids a person to perform an act or pursue a treatment which he or she honestly believes to be right, the person may break or ignore the law. They may genuinely consider the prohibition as unjust. The fact that the law was reached by a democratic procedure does not make it a just solution[33]. In most cases, the democratic decision-making is a fair way of achieving a compromise between competing claims[32], but that does not mean that every law voted by a democratically elected parliament ought to be obeyed.

Whether or not cross-border reproductive care can be seen as civil disobedience depends on the definition one adopts. According to Raz, civil disobedience 'is a politically motivated breach of law designed either to contribute directly to a change of a law or of a public policy or to express one's protest against, or dissociation from, a law or public policy'[33]. However, there is no agreement on when an act qualifies as civil disobedience. It has been argued, for instance, that the person committing the act should have the intention to change the law. It is not clear whether cross-border traveling is performed with this intention. Perhaps it would be more appropriate to call it 'evasive non-compliance'[34]. By traveling, patients indicate that they do not intend to abide by the law and do not want to suffer the negative consequences of the law. Openness has also been proposed as a condition for civil disobedience. If all Italian couples who seek treatment abroad would tell their friends and family, this would most likely have an large impact on the general perception of the law. However, infertility is not just medical treatment; it is a highly personal and emotional problem. It is unreasonable to expect couples who need recourse to donor gametes to tell their friends and acquaintances. Another commonly stated condition to determine whether an act is one of civil disobedience is that lawful alternatives for changing the law or policy have been exhausted[35]. The referendum held in Italy can be seen as a legal attempt to over-turn parts of the law. Since it failed (not surprisingly, given the condition that 50% of the electorate should cast their vote for it to be valid), no other options are available. Still, it suffices to look at the attention given to cross-border reproductive care to realize that there is strong pressure emanating from such movements on the existing law. The same mechanism occurred in a number of countries regarding the abortion laws. When citizens leave a country in large numbers to avoid a law, this is embarrassing for the government and an incitement to make amendments.

CONCLUSION

Cross-border reproductive care is sure to increase in the coming years. Globalization also takes place in the provision of health-care services. The great-est danger created by these movements is fraud, and violations of the rules of good clinical practice. Purely commercial clinics operating without adequate control are almost certainly going to cut down on expenses for safety. An independent inter-national system should be established which accredits competent and safe clinics. Simultaneously, however, efforts should be made to reduce the number of people traveling. This obligation is generated by the considerable risks and dangers that this type of traveling may generate. The two main mechanisms to reach this goal are a flexible law on medically assisted reproduction and a reduction of the costs of infertility treatment by means of insurance coverage and/or public funding.

REFERENCES

1. Inspectie voor de Gezondheidszorg. Jaarrapportage 2002 van de Wet Afbreking Zwangerschap. Den Haag: Inspectie voor de Gezondheidszorg, 2003.
2. Pennings G. Legal harmonization and reproductive tourism in Europe. Hum Reprod 2004; 19: 2689–94.
3. Matorras R. Reproductive exile versus reproductive tourism [Letter]. Hum Reprod 2005; 20: 3571.
4. Commission of the European Communities. Follow-up to the high level reflection process on patient mobility and healthcare developments in the European Union. Brussels: Commission of the European Communities, 2004.
5. Martin N. Website bypasses sperm donor law. The Daily Telegraph 30 March 2005.
6. Papps N. Rush for designer babies. The Sunday Mail 5 September 2004.
7. Kilani Z. Controversies in gender selection. Presented at the 18th World Congress on Fertility and Sterility, IFFS, Montreal, Canada, May 2004.
8. Vandervorst M, Staessen C, Sermon K, et al. The Brussels' experience of more than 5 years of clinical preimplantation genetic diagnosis. Hum Reprod Update 2000; 6: 364–73.

9.   Pennings G. Measuring the welfare of the child: in search of the appropriate evaluation principle. Hum Reprod 1999; 14: 1146–50.

10. Hervey TK. Buy baby: the European Union and regulation of human reproduction. Ox J Legal Stud 1998; 8: 207–33.

11. Henn W. Genetic screening with the DNA chip: a new Pandora's box? J Med Ethics 1999; 25: 200–3.

12. Brazier M. Regulating the reproduction business? Med Law Rev 1999; 7: 166–93.

13. Millns S. Reproducing inequalities: assisted conception and the challenge of legal pluralism. J Soc Welfare Fam Law 2002; 24: 19–36.

14. Engelhardt HT Jr. The Foundations of Bioethics. New York: Oxford University Press, 1986.

15. Den Hartogh G. Should we welcome supranational regulation of bioethical issues? In Royal Netherlands Academy of Arts and Science, eds. Bioethics and Health in International Context. Amsterdam: Royal Netherlands Academy of Arts and Science, 2002: 37–44.

16. United Nations General Assembly. Letter dated 2 April 2003 from the Permanent Representative of Costa Rica to the United Nations addressed to the Secretary-General, fifty-eighth session A/58/73, 2003.

17. Human Genetics Alert. Appendix 30. Memorandum from Human Genetics Alert. The United Kingdom Parliament, Select Committee on Science and Technology. 2003, www.publications.parliament.uk/pa/cm200304/cmselect/cmsctech/599/599 we31.htm.

18. Stafford N. Stem cell collaboration illegal. The Scientist, 31 August 2004. www.the-scientist.com/news/20040831/04.

19. Kreimer SF. The law of choice and choice of law: abortion, the right to travel, and extraterritorial regulation in American federalism. NY Univ Law Rev 1992; 67: 451–519.

20. Magureanu G. Egg donation and conflict within the Romanian legal framework. Presented at Core European Seminar: Human Egg Trading and the Exploitation of Women, Brussels, 30 June 2005.

21. Gurmankin AD. Risk information provided to prospective oocyte donors in preliminary phone call. Am J Bioethics 2001; 1: 3–13.

22. Emery M. What ethical issues on the welfare of the child need to be addressed during psychological counselling? Presented at Pre-congress course – Joint SIG Psychology and Counselling and Ethics and Law, European Society of Human Reproduction and Embryology, 19 June 2005, Copenhagen, Denmark.

23. Global Egg Donation Resource What we can do for you. www.gedr.com/info.asp. Accessed June 1, 2005.

24. Ferrando G. Artificial insemination in Italy. In Evans D, ed. Creating the Child. The Hague: Martinus Nijhoff Publishers, 1996: 255–66.

25. Bell J, Stroh M. U.S. science tested on humans abroad. The Baltimore Sun, 17 October 2003.

26. Reagan LJ. Crossing the border for abortions: California activists, Mexican clinics, and the creation of a feminist health agency in the 1960s. Fem Stud 2000; 26: 323–48.

27. Hermans HEGM. Cross-border health care in the European Union: recent legal implications of Decker and Kohll. J Eval Clin Pract 2000; 6: 431–9.

28. Kostakopoulou D. Ideas, norms and European citizenship: explaining institutional change. Mod Law Rev 2005; 68: 233–67.

29. Conseil Fédéral Suisse. Avis du conseil fédéral. Initiative 'pour une procréation respectant la dignité humaine'. 2000; www.admin.ch/f/pore/va/20000312/explic/index.html.

30. Benagiano G, Gianaroli L. The new Italian IVF legislation. Reprod Biomed Online 2004; 9: 117–25.

31. Gordijn B. Regulating moral dissent in an open society: the Dutch experience with pragmatic tolerance. J Med Philos 2001; 26: 225–44.

32. Singer P. Disobedience as a plea for reconsiderations. In Bedau HA, ed. Civil Disobedience in Focus. London: Routledge Press, 1991: 122–9.

33. Raz J. The Authority of Law: Essays on Law and Morality. Oxford: Clarendon Press, 1979.

34. Childress JF. Civil disobedience, conscientious objection, and evasive noncompliance: a framework for the analysis and assessment of illegal actions in health care. J Med Philos 1985; 10: 63–83.

35. Greenawalt K. Justifying nonviolent disobedience. In Bedau HA, ed. Civil Disobedience in Focus. London: Routledge, 1991: 170–88.

Chapter 5

Risking parenthood?
Serious viral illness, parenting and
the welfare of the child

Carole Gilling-Smith

INTRODUCTION

In vitro techniques and human immunodeficiency virus (HIV) evolved as medical challenges during the same era. The first brought hope and life to couples struggling with subfertility. The second led to a global viral epidemic and brought misery and death to millions of young people of reproductive age. Two decades on, advances in both areas have produced the ethical dilemma of assisting reproduction in patients infected with HIV and other potentially life-threatening viral illnesses such as hepatitis C (HCV). The development of effective antiretroviral (ARV) regimens, together with the sharp drop in vertical transmission risk for HIV, has changed the reproductive limitations that these serious viral diseases once posed. As a result there has been a sharp rise in the number of HIV-infected men and women looking to reproductive specialists for advice on how to conceive safely. In this chapter, we analyze the role of assisted reproduction in patients with potentially life-threatening viral illnesses, in particular HIV, the ethical implications of offering such treatment for the patient, the uninfected partner and the unborn child and the risks to non-infected patients being treated within the same fertility center.

HIV: A CHANGED DISEASE

HIV affects over 39 million people worldwide, of whom 37 million are adults and just under half are women[1]. The majority of those living with HIV are of reproductive age, and young people (age 15–24) account for half of all new HIV infections. Advances in ARV regimens over the past 10 years have transformed the natural course of the disease by slowing down, and in the majority of cases effectively aborting, the virus's ability to destroy the immune system, leading to the acquired immunodeficiency syndrome (AIDS). Over 20 million people have died of AIDS since 1981, and in underdeveloped countries, where access to ARVs is at present limited due to cost, the disease continues to cause high fatalities. In these areas, reproduction is strongly discouraged, although strong cultural pressures lead many to ignore government and medical advice on this matter, which further fuels the global epidemic. However, a place for reproduction is emerging in the developed world where infected patients receive close monitoring of their disease, and effective ARV treatment can be started promptly once viral load rises and CD4 count falls below a critical level. For these patients, provided that they are adhering to their treatment, HIV is now defined as a chronic, not fatal, disease. Life expectancy from the time of diagnosis improves with younger age (< 50 years), CD4 count > 200, low or undetectable viral load and the absence of previous AIDS-related symptoms. Co-infection with HCV, which is often seen in HIV acquired following transfusion of blood products, e.g. in hemophiliacs, or in previous intravenous drug abuse, carries a worse prognosis. An infected individual with a negative viral load and CD4 count > 200 is currently estimated to be able to remain free of AIDS-related symptoms for at least 20 years from diagnosis, provided that he adheres to therapy, which is usually a complex combination of ARVs that are varied from time to time to prevent viral resistance developing.

A second significant advance in HIV management over the past decade has been the reduction in mother-to-child transmission (MCT) risk from 15–35%[2] to below 2% through the use of ARVs, particularly during the third trimester and delivery, avoidance of breast-feeding and a carefully timed and planned delivery[3]. Cesarean section, once the only form of delivery for positive women, is not always necessary[4]. The combination of better life quality and expectancy, together with reduced MCT risk, has led to a reanalysis of the reproductive status of HIV individuals and their partners and their right to have children[5–10].

HEPATITIS B AND C

Hepatitis B virus (HBV) is not generally regarded as serious a viral illness as HIV. It is, however, a major cause of chronic hepatitis, cirrhosis and hepatocellular cancer worldwide, and MCT accounts for over 40% of cases of chronic infection. Sexual transmission risk is twice as high as for HIV. From an ethical point of view, the main difference from HIV and HCV is that an effective vaccine exists, and the uninfected partner, newborn and health workers can be protected. The main concern with HBV in reproductive medicine is ensuring that samples from patients who are HBV antigen positive are handled in a separate laboratory, and strict protocols for handling high-risk samples are in place[11].

HCV infection is the leading cause of liver disease in the world, with 20% of patients developing cirrhosis within 20 years of infection. Many of these will progress to hepatocellular carcinoma. The majority of patients are infected through parenteral spread (blood products, shared needles, needle-stick injury). Sexual transmission risk is very low unless the patient is co-infected with HIV. Unlike HBV, there is no vaccine for HCV, and sperm washing is advisable in discordant couples where the male is infected[12]. Hepatitis C is not affected by, and does not influence, the normal course of pregnancy. MCT risk depends on whether the mother is HCV-RNA-positive or -negative. If she is HCV antibody-positive but HCV-RNA-negative, the risk is < 1%, but increases to 11% if she is HCV-RNA-positive and 16% if she is co-infected with HIV[13]. HCV-RNA-positive men and women are usually advised to receive treatment with interferon-α and/or ribavirin treatment, to reduce viral load prior to assisted conception. In both instances the treatment has to be stopped 6 months pre-conceptually because of potential mutagenic effects of these drugs on the fetus. There are no other specific measures available to protect the neonate, as immunoglobulins confer no added protection and a vaccine is not available. HCV does not appear to be transmitted during breast-feeding.

THE WELFARE OF THE CHILD AND SERIOUS VIRAL ILLNESS

A distinction has to be made between two scenarios. The first is where infected patients make their own choice about whether or not to have children and do not involve a reproductive specialist. Here, to a certain extent, the welfare of the future child rests in their own hands, as they make the final decision on whether or not it is appropriate for them to become parents. Pre-conceptual counseling from their physician or health adviser should form an integral part of specialist care so that they can make an informed decision. Issues such as options to reduce MCT risk and horizontal transmission risk to the uninfected partner should be discussed, and support networks in the event of the infected partner becoming seriously ill or dying explored. The second scenario is where infected patients seek the help of a reproductive specialist to overcome fertility issues and/or minimize sexual transmission risk. It is the latter scenario which poses, in many cases, difficult ethical dilemmas for the reproductive specialist and his team.

In deciding whether or not to treat an HIV-infected couple, the reproductive specialist has to take into consideration the four major underlying principles of medical ethics: non-maleficence (doing no harm), beneficence (doing good), respecting autonomy and justice (providing honest and fair care)[14,15]. This has to be done in the context of the infected individual, the uninfected partner and the future child, and society as a whole.

Consideration of the welfare of the child remains a fundamental step in preparing any couple for assisted conception. In the UK it is still a legal requirement under the Human Fertilisation and Embryology (HFE) Act (1990) to seek written confirmation from the patient's general practitioner that there are no issues that might affect the welfare of the unborn child or the need for that child to have a father. The reproductive specialist has to consider carefully the environment into which a child may be born and ensure that it is adequate for its physical and psychological growth and development. HIV and HCV, particularly in individuals who are co-infected, have important welfare-of-the-child implications aside from MCT.

Infected patients may have acquired their illness through a life-style which threatens the safety of their uninfected partner and future child if it is maintained, e.g. intravenous drug abuse and prostitution. In addition, controlling their disease is complex and requires their cooperation and motivation and, when reproduction is envisaged, their agreement to involve a multidisciplinary team including a reproductive specialist, HIV physician and, in the case of the infected female, HIV specialist obstetrician, and to comply with advice given. In practical terms, assessing the welfare of the child in patients with a viral illness has to involve the multidisciplinary team, who have far greater insight into the potential risks of offering treatment in any individual case than does the patient's general practitioner.

Assessment of the welfare of the child forms the backbone in the process of decision-making in patients with serious viral illnesses and encompasses the following factors:

(1) Horizontal transmission risk to the uninfected partner;

(2) MCT risk;

(3) Potential teratogenic risk of ARVs;

(4) Life expectancy of the infected individual;

(5) Patient compliance;

(6) High-risk behavior and life-style issues;

(7) Support network if the infected individual becomes seriously ill or dies.

The decision of whether or not to offer treatment has to be individualized once all these issues have been carefully considered and the patient has received appropriate reproductive counseling.

Horizontal transmission risk to the uninfected partner

In doing no harm, the first consideration is to ensure that the risks of viral transmission to the uninfected partner and unborn child are addressed. If a couple, where one or both partners are infected with a serious virus, are denied access to assisted reproductive techniques, will they have a higher or lower risk of infecting their partner or child? The conditions differ for HIV and HCV, and when the male, as opposed to the female, is infected.

The risk of sexual transmission of HIV from an infected male to an uninfected female is quoted at 0.1–0.5% per act of unprotected intercourse[16], provided that the couple are in a stable monogamous relationship, not abusing intravenous drugs or participating in any other form of high-risk activity. A child cannot become infected unless the mother becomes infected first. In the absence of an effective vaccine for HIV, couples are currently advised to avoid unprotected intercourse at all times. Viral load in semen correlates poorly with that in serum[17], and men with undetectable plasma HIV viral levels, such as those on antiretrovirals, can still transmit HIV in semen[18].

Unfortunately, there is a widely held belief amongst HIV-infected men on anti-retroviral medication, with an undetectable viral load, that unprotected intercourse limited to the fertile window is a safe and acceptable method of conceiving. In a retrospective study of 77 discordant couples attempting to conceive, in whom the HIV-positive male partner was on antiretrovirals and had had undetectable HIV for at least 6 months, no seroconversions were noted[19]. This study made no attempt to analyze seroconversions in couples who failed to conceive, and, overall, numbers are too small to draw any valid conclusions on the safety of this approach. There is only one prospective study which has analyzed the risk of viral transmission in discordant couples trying to conceive using carefully timed unprotected intercourse. Four women from a cohort of 92 HIV-negative women with HIV-positive partners seroconverted, although these seroconversions were related to inconsistent condom use post-conception[20]. Recently published guidelines on the subject in the UK recommend that HIV-discordant couples where the male partner is infected, who wish to conceive and eliminate or significantly reduce HIV transmission risk to their uninfected partner, should consider either sperm washing with insemination or donor insemination[4,13,21]. Donor sperm is screened for HIV and other viral infections, and this effectively removes all risk of viral transmission to the uninfected partner or child. However, this approach takes away the possibility of the infected parent having a genetic link to his offspring, which in itself carries numerous emotional and psychological sequelae, particularly in an individual with a life-threatening viral illness. Sperm washing is a method of processing semen in a density gradient, which removes HIV from the seminal fluid and non-sperm cells and relies on the observation, well supported in the literature, that HIV does not attach itself to spermatozoa[22]. The technique was pioneered in the late 1980s and first results published in 1992[23]. The female partner is inseminated with the infected partner's 'washed' sperm at the fertile time of her cycle. A sensitive HIV assay (nucleic acid-based sequence amplification or similar commercial assay) is carried out on an aliquot of the processed semen prior to this being used in treatment as an internal control. Some 5% of samples have detectable virus post-processing and cannot be used[13]. The technique can be combined with other assisted conception methods such as IVF if fertility factors are also present. It is important to appreciate that the technique is a *risk-reduction* and not *risk-free* method, and virus could still be present in the washed sample at a titer below the detection limit of the HIV assay (e.g. 25 viral copies/10^6 sperm). Over the past 5 years there has been a steady increase in the number of centers in Europe and America able to offer this technique. A European database of results recently published is reassuring, with no seroconversions in either the uninfected partner or the child in 4989 cycles of sperm washing performed, resulting in the birth of over 500 healthy HIV-negative children[24]. The main limitation to this technique is access and funding. At present, sperm washing is only available at a few clinics throughout the world (20 centers in Europe and one in the USA), and in the majority of cases is not state funded. Adoption is an alternative to sperm washing or donor insemination for these couples, but remains at present a very limited option for HIV-concordant and -discordant couples. Most agencies regard HIV infection in the parent as a significant undesirable factor when assessing the suitability of parents requesting to adopt. So, for the infected male, sperm washing and donor insemination can reduce viral transmission risk to the uninfected partner and child over and above timed intercourse, and on that basis the reproductive physician has an obligation to discuss these options, and their pros and cons, with the couple even if other welfare-of-the-child issues become apparent and lead to the couple being refused treatment.

Transmission risk from infected female to uninfected male is lower at 0.05% per act of unprotected intercourse. In couples where the female partner alone is positive, current guidelines recommend self-insemination of the partner's ejaculated sperm into the vagina using quills at the fertile time of the month[4]. When both partners are positive they are advised to consider insemination of the female partner using washed sperm, as there is a small risk of one partner re-infecting the other with a different strain of HIV, a process referred to as superinfection (exposure to different ARVs can lead to viral mutation). Fertility, particularly tubal, appears to be reduced in HIV-positive women based on retrospective data from the developing[25] and developed world[26] and prospective data[27] from the UK. It is important, therefore, to ensure that couples failing to conceive with attempts are referred for fertility investigations after 6–12 months of attempts and offered assisted reproduction such as IVF if appropriate. Failure to do so increases the risk of the uninfected partner becoming infected, as the couple are likely to attempt to increase their chances of conceiving by having unprotected intercourse[28]. It may well be that, after appropriate counseling and evaluation of the welfare-of-the-child issues, proceeding to offering treatment is not in the best interest of the unborn child, but access to reproductive assistance should not be denied at the outset[29] The principles of autonomy and doing no harm are in this way respected.

MCT risk

Mother-to-child transmission of HIV can only be significantly decreased if the patient has access to a multidisciplinary approach, which includes pre-conceptual counseling and close monitoring during pregnancy and postnatally. In addition, the newborn needs close pediatric monitoring and a short course of ARVs. It is not appropriate to offer reproductive assistance if these conditions cannot be met with any certainty, because the patient either refuses to be monitored or does not comply with advice given (see below), or where access to specialist obstetric care is not possible. The reproductive physician has a duty, therefore, to liaise closely with the patient's HIV physician and obstetrician to ensure that optimal ARV medication is used and that the patient is adhering to the suggested regimen of drugs. In the case of HCV-RNA-positive women, it is strongly advisable to defer pregnancy until a course of interferon-α and/or ribavirin has been given, as this will significantly reduce the risk of MCT. There are cases, however, when deferring treatment to complete a course of interferon, for example, may be in conflict with maximizing a woman's chances of conceiving as she enters the period of accelerated ovarian decline in her late 30s.

Increased MCT risk has for a long time been used to deny women with HIV or HCV infection access to reproductive care. As awareness of MCT risk when appropriate interventions are used increases, the arguments for denying treatment fade. How can one justify denying IVF to women with HIV and a < 2% risk of MCT when it is acceptable to treat women with congenital heart disease or cystic fibrosis, which confer a 20% risk of the offspring being affected, or women with insulin-dependent diabetes, who have a 2% risk of their child being affected[7,29]? Many women in their early to mid-40s are offered assisted conception, and their risk of giving birth to a child with trisomy 21 is significantly higher than 2%, as not all will opt for prenatal testing.

Potential teratogenic risk of ARVs

Antiretroviral drugs are potent drugs, and for many there are no guarantees that teratogenesis will not occur. Zidovudine (AZT) is well tried and tested in pregnancy and appears to be safe and highly effective, and is the only antiretroviral agent currently licensed for use in pregnancy in the UK. There are limited data for most ARVs, although some nucleosides (such as tenofovir) fall into category B as opposed to category C by virtue of animal study results.

Life expectancy of the infected individual

In the past it was argued that patients with HIV should not parent because of their reduced life expectancy. As previously discussed, this argument no longer stands. The new argument is that it is not reasonable to offer assisted reproduction to patients with a high viral load, low CD4 count or resistant disease, and that treatment can only be justified in the presence of 'stable' disease. A CD4 count > 400 and undetectable viral load has been proposed as an arbitrary definition of 'stable' disease. There are many examples where a patient may be 'stable' by these criteria but develop HIV-related complications during the course of treatment, for example a patient who develops lymphoma or another tumor as a recognized complication of HIV. Does this preclude them from treatment in the future if they return for treatment when in remission? Likewise, a patient's CD4 count may fluctuate over a short space of time, particularly if there is a switch in medication, so one cannot make too hard and fast rules. It is clear, however, that a woman with AIDS-related symptoms and poorly controlled disease resistant to safe ARV regimens should be discouraged from parenting as her life expectancy is likely to be poor, and she may need to take potentially teratogenic drugs in the first trimester of pregnancy to control her symptoms.

Probably the most contentious area in the whole ethical debate about providing reproductive care to those with serious viral illness is the situation of the concordant couple in the case of HIV or where both parents have a serious viral illness. A recent European Society of Human Reproduction and Embryology (ESHRE) Taskforce on the ethics of offering assisted conception to those infected with HIV recommended that medical assistance should be restricted to serodiscordant couples until there was clearer evidence that life expectancy for those with symptomatic disease was improved[9]. With the reclassification of HIV as a chronic disease, the time has come to challenge this view. At present there are no published guidelines to define who should or should not be offered reproductive care, and it is left to the individual physician to tease out the risks and benefits of offering treatment after careful analysis of the life expectancy of each potential parent. Other welfare-of-the-child issues such as life-style, high-risk behavior and compliance with medical treatment need to be taken into consideration. Nothing in life can be assured, but a statistical expectation of at least one parent being able to see the child through to adulthood would seem a reasonable argument to proceed with offering reproductive assistance. HIV is unfortunately a disease which still stigmatizes the affected individual and leads to discrimination in many aspects of life – the medical field being no exception. It is important, therefore, that reproductive physicians view HIV in the same light as other serious medical conditions with similar life expectancies, and do not let themselves become prejudiced. Many couples are considered suitable candidates for reproductive care, despite clear indications of declining health and possible reduced life expectancy in both parents. A common example is the obese couple who smoke and lead an unhealthy life-style, which puts them both at high risk of developing early-onset cardiovascular disease. Less common is the situation where each prospective parent has a chronic physical or mental disease such as diabetes or schizophrenia, or a genetically increased risk of developing cancer, e.g. familial polyposis coli. These situations do not automatically bar the way to medical assistance to procreate, but are treated on a case-by-case basis.

Patient compliance

It is evident that the reproductive specialist cannot offer treatment to a couple where there is clear evidence of non-compliance to medication or advice. Not only is the potential life expectancy of the individual potentially compromised if ARVs are not taken, but, more pertinent, in the positive female one is relying on her adhering to a strict regimen of combination therapy in the third trimester and during labor to minimize MCT. Likewise, for men who are in a discordant relationship, who fail to practice safe sex and put their partner and unborn child at risk, it is questionable whether such couples should be offered sperm washing.

High-risk behavior and life-style issues

A significant proportion of men living with HIV are in same-sex relationships, and many are looking at the possibility of fathering through insemination of their washed sperm into a suitable and willing female friend. Such women are often themselves in same-sex relationships, and complexities arise as to who will actually bring up the child if the male and female partner are not in any form of relationship. This is where consideration for the welfare of the child becomes the most important deciding factor in offering treatment. Whilst the demand for this approach is rising, tight ethical guidelines have, to date, precluded same-sex couples with HIV from proceeding to treatment.

Support network if the infected individual becomes seriously ill or dies

The importance of pre-conceptual counseling in the management of these patients has already been discussed. One aspect that needs to be explored with the couple both individually and together is the support available to the partner and future child if the infected parent becomes seriously ill or dies. This is in fact an issue that all prospective parents should explore, but in reality it falls on their own initiative to do so. In the context of serious viral illness, the probability of a parent dying is far higher, and the reproductive physician has an obligation to ensure that the couple explore the specific measures they would take and, if appropriate, involve family and friends. Many HIV-positive women living in developed countries are from sub-Saharan Africa, but the men in these relationships are often financially tied to working in Africa. In the context of parenthood, the future mother may be effectively a single parent and be expected to cope alone with her illness and a young child.

RISKS OF IVF/ICSI IN WOMEN WITH HIV

In being mindful of the basic ethical tenet of doing no harm, the reproductive physician needs to evaluate the risks of the invasive procedures used in IVF treatments for the fetus of a seropositive mother. The numbers of positive women treated to date are small[30,31], and there is a paucity of data on safety. Needling the ovary to collect oocytes and transferring embryos to the uterus are invasive procedures which may expose the oocyte or embryo to HIV. Whether or not this is sufficient to infect the fetus at an early developmental stage and lead to the birth of a positive child is an unknown but theoretical possibility. There is good evidence that HIV is present in both follicular fluid and endometrial samples of positive women, irrespective of viral load[32]. For this reason, reproductive physicians offering positive women assisted reproduction should ensure that pregnancy outcome and HIV status of the child are recorded in all cases, as it is important to define whether IVF or intracytoplasmic sperm injection (ICSI) could lead to an increase in MCT rates over and above those observed after natural conception.

VIRAL TRANSMISSION RISK TO OTHER PATIENTS ATTENDING THE TREATMENT CENTER

A major concern in providing treatment to patients with a blood-borne viral illness is the potential for viral transmission to non-infected patients, and contamination of their gametes and embryos. In terms of non-maleficence, reproductive physicians have a responsibility for ensuring that uninfected patients attending the same center, as well as staff, are not put at risk. Unfortunately, there are no published guidelines on the subject, only recommendations[11,13]. Nosocomial contamination between patients has been described for HIV, HCV and HBV, and cross-contamination in tanks storing biological material has also been clearly demonstrated. In the UK, the Human Fertilisation and Embryology Authority (HFEA) has endorsed separate cryostorage of gametes and embryos for each viral infection or infection combination. This has an appreciable cost implication, but unfortunately it is one which will have to be borne out by the small number of clinics prepared to offer infected patients treatment. In Europe, many centers have moved to the universal use of heat-sealed straws, which have been shown to be effective in minimizing viral transmission risk during cryostorage[11]. Another concern is where and how samples are collected and handled. Standard operating procedures need to be reviewed to minimize the risk of cross-contamination. It is recommended that laboratory procedures on infected samples are separated in either time and/or space from those carried out on screen-negative samples. The latter is best addressed by developing a separate laboratory designed to handle potentially contaminated material[11]. It is assumed that universal precautions are used at all times. These added measures serve to minimize risk further, reassure non-infected patients and protect the service from medicolegal action in the event of a patient becoming infected following treatment. In the USA, the cost implications of building a separate laboratory and providing separate cryostorage have been used as a reason to deny HIV-positive women access to assisted conception[6], which is in fact in contradiction to the revised policy recently published by the American Society for Reproductive Medicine, which advocates non-discrimination[29]. Clearly these requirements are costly, and will only service a small proportion of the total population. The most rational and cost-effective approach is to develop a limited number of specialized treatment centers for patients with blood-borne viral illnesses, which should be strategically placed geographically.

OVUM DONATION IN THE HIV-POSITIVE PATIENT

Assisted reproduction in the case of the female patient with a serious viral illness may involve a fourth party in cases where ovum donation is deemed appropriate. This adds a new dimension to the ethical challenge. Women who choose to donate eggs do so for many reasons, but it would seem reasonable for a potential egg donor to be made aware of a recipient's viral status, as this may affect her decision to proceed. The unknown risks of IVF in HIV-positive women together with the potential of the child being born infected are clear indications for in-depth pre-conceptual counseling of both donor and recipient.

Two recent studies of positive women undergoing IVF in Spain suggest that HIV-positive women have lower pregnancy rates than HIV-negative controls[31]. These differences are not observed in HIV-positive women undergoing ovum donation, pointing towards an effect of HIV ovarian reserve rather than endometrial receptivity. These figures suggest that positive women may increasingly turn to ovum donation if they fail to conceive successfully with their own gametes.

CONCLUSION

Reproductive specialists are duty bound to prevent harm and do good to society as a whole. Much of the above discussion has focused on the individual: the patient and, in particular, the welfare of the prospective child. In the wider context, reducing horizontal and vertical transmission risk through appropriate medical care is of long-term benefit to society, particularly at a time when heterosexual transmission rates for HIV are rising[1]. Offering reproductive care has to be carefully balanced against the risk of increasing the burden on society of children born into difficult social circumstances, and either being infected themselves or being orphaned at a young age.

Although not a legal body, the American Society for Reproductive Medicine Ethics Committee stated in 2004 that 'unless health care workers can show that they lack the skills and facilities to treat HIV-positive patients safely or that the patient refused reasonable testing and treatment, they may be legally as well as ethically obligated to provide requested reproductive assistance'[29]. Article 12 of the European Court of Human Rights states that 'men and women of marriageable age have the right to marry and found a family, according to the national laws governing the exercise of this right'. Although individuals with serious viral illness and in particular HIV-concordant couples should continue to be carefully evaluated in ethical and psychosocial terms on a case-by-case basis, they have rights. Reproductive physicians therefore need to be mindful of the possibility of legal action being taken against them if they do not have robust arguments for denying infected patients treatment.

REFERENCES

1. UNAIDS. Report on the global AIDS epidemic. Geneva: Joint United Nations Programme on HIV/AIDS (UNAIDS), 2004.
2. Newell M. The natural history of vertically acquired HIV infection: the European Collaborative Study. J Perinat Med 1991; 19: S257–62.
3. European Collaborative Study. Mother to child transmission of HIV infection in the era of highly active antiretroviral therapy. Clin Infect Dis 2005; 40: 458–65.

4.   Hawkins D, Blott M, Clayden P, et al. Guidelines for the management of HIV infection in pregnant women and the prevention of mother-to-child transmission of HIV. HIV Med 2005; 6 (Suppl 2): 107–48.

5.   Ryan KJ. Using metaphor to deal with human immunodeficiency infection and infertility. Fertil Steril 2001; 75: 859–60.

6.   Sauer MV. Providing fertility care to those with HIV: time to re-examine healthcare policy. Am J Bioethics 2003; 3: 33–40.

7.   Gilling-Smith C, Smith JR, Semprini AE. HIV and infertility: time to treat. There's no justification for denying treatment to parents who are HIV positive. Br Med J 2001; 322: 566–7.

8.   Englert Y, Van Vooren JP, Place I, et al. ART in HIV-infected couples. Has the time come for a change in attitude? Hum Reprod 2001; 16: 1309–15.

9.   The ESHRE Ethics and Law Task Force. Taskforce 8: ethics of medically assisted fertility treatment for HIV positive men and women. Hum Reprod 2004; 19: 2454–6.

10. Minkoff H, Santoro N. Ethical considerations in the treatment of infertility in women with human immunodeficiency virus infection. N Engl J Med 2000; 342: 1748–50.

11. Gilling-Smith C, Emiliani S, Almeida P, et al. Laboratory safety during assisted reproduction in patients with blood-borne viruses. Hum Reprod 2005; 20: 1433–8.

12. Pasquier C, Daudin M, Righi L, et al. Sperm washing and virus nucleic acid detection to reduce HIV and hepatitis C virus transmission in serodiscordant couples wishing to have children. AIDS 2000; 14: 2093–9.

13. Gilling-Smith C, Almeida P. HIV, hepatitis B and hepatitis C and infertility: reducing risk. Hum Fertil (Camb) 2003; 6: 106–12.

14. Sharma S, Gilling-Smith C, Semprini AE, et al. View 1: assisted conception in couples with HIV infection. Sex Transm Infect 2003; 79: 185–8.

15. Beauchamp TL, Childress JF. Principles of Biomedical Ethics, 4th edn. New York: Oxford University Press, 1994.

16. Gray RH, Wawer MJ, Brookmeyer R, et al. Probability of HIV-1 transmission per coital act in monogamous, heterosexual, HIV-1 serodiscordant couples in Rakai, Uganda. Lancet 2003; 357: 1149–53.

17. Luizzi G, Chirianni A, Clement M, et al. Analysis of HIV-1 load in blood, semen and saliva: evidence for different viral compartments in a cross-sectional and longitudinal study. AIDS 1996; 10: F51–56.

18. Zhang H, Domadula G, Beumont M, et al. Human immunodeficiency virus type 1 in the semen of men receiving highly active antiretroviral therapy. N Engl J Med 1998; 339: 1803–9.

19. Barreiro P, Soriano V, Nunez M, Gonzalez-Lanoz J. Benefit of antiretroviral therapy for serodiscordant couples willing to be parents. Presented at the 7th International Congress on Drug Therapy in HIV Infection, Glasgow, Scotland, November 2004.

20. Mandelbrot L, Heard I, Henrion-Geant R, Henrion R. Natural conception in HIV-negative women with HIV-infected partners. Lancet 1997; 349: 850–1.

21. Semprini AE, Vucetich A, Hollander L. Sperm washing, use of HAART and role of elective Caesarean section. Curr Opin Obstet Gynecol 2004; 16: 465–70.

22. Gilling-Smith C. HIV prevention. Assisted reproduction in HIV-discordant couples. AIDS Read 2000; 10: 581–7.

23. Semprini AE, Levi-Setti P, Bozzo M, et al. Insemination of HIV-negative women with processed semen of HIV-positive partners. Lancet 1992; 340: 1317–19.

24. Semprini AE, Fiore S. HIV and reproduction. Curr Opin Obstet Gynecol 2004; 16: 257–62.

25. Glynn J, Buve A, Carael M, et al. Decreased fertility among HIV-1 infected women attending antenatal clinics in three African cities. JAIDS 2000; 25: 345–52.

26. Thackway S, Furner V, Mijch A, et al. Fertility and reproductive choice in women with HIV-1 infection. AIDS 1997; 11: 663–7.

27. Frodsham L, Boag F, Barton S, Gilling-Smith C. HIV positive fertility care for couples in in the UK – supply and demand. Fertil Steril 2005; in press.

28. Frodsham LC, Smith JR, Gilling-Smith C. Assessment of welfare of the child in HIV positive couples. Hum Reprod 2004; 19: 2420–3.

29. ASRM Ethics Committee. Human immunodeficiency virus and infertility treatment. Fertil Steril 2004; 82 (Suppl 1): S228–31.

30. Ohl J, Partisani M, Wittemer C, et al. Assisted reproduction techniques for HIV serodiscordant couples: 18 months of experience. Hum Reprod 2003; 18: 1244–9.

31. Coll O, Suy A, Vernaeve V, et al. Associated factors to the low reproductive outcome in infertile HIV-infected women. Hum Reprod 2005; 20 (Suppl 1): 20–2.

32. Frodsham LCG, Cox AD, Almeida PA, et al. In vitro fertilisation in HIV positive women: risk of mother to embryo viral transmission. Hum Reprod 2004; 9: 138.

PART III

THE OFFSPRING
AND SOCIETY AT LARGE

Chapter 6

The welfare of the child:
whose responsibility?

Françoise Shenfield and Claude Sureau

When would-be parents do not require our assistance, they may not need to justify their decision of conception to anyone else than to each other, and even then sometimes only at a subconscious level. Their privacy may be invaded by family and friends when they discuss the matter, but unless one of them has a serious medical condition, they would generally not ask 'leave to reproduce' from a physician. 'The reasons they wish to have children and the conditions in which they intend to raise them concern their private life'[1].

The nature of and means to achieve this private-life decision to procreate has taken a quantum leap from chance to a planned decision in the past 40–50 years, thanks to the better survival of neonates and children, wider and easier availability of contraception, antenatal screening and safe terminations of pregnancy. Any form of planning implies intention, and means responsibility for the outcome. Because our patients have to request help and agree (or not) to a mode of treatment, this means that reflection about this responsibility is necessarily given more time than for the five in six couples who do not require our help, even if many planned pregnancies where there is no fertility problem also entail a thoughtful reflection about the future child. But the very fact that a third party is not normally implicated by this concern for the welfare of the future child has been used as an argument by those who disapprove of the legal requirement in the UK to take into account the 'the welfare of the child born from licensed treatment'[2]: a recent parliamentary committee report has criticized this legal phrasing, judging that taking into account the welfare of the child must always be the consequence of 'prejudice'[3]. Many clinicians and ethicists, however, feel that it is part of our professional responsibility to do so[4,5].

In general, a reproductive decision is still mostly taken in private, unless the social context fails women by not providing their legally enshrined rights to contraception or termination of pregnancy for instance, or unless they live in societies where this is not available. When a pregnancy is established, men do not generally have rights to prevent their partner having a termination[6], but when they plan a pregnancy together, and especially ask a third party (the medical profession) to assist, the responsibility is shared from that moment to ensure that the future child's welfare is considered. This applies also if they are fertile and wish to avoid extra risk, as in couples with human immunodeficiency virus (HIV), when sperm washing not only benefits the seronegative woman whose partner is seropositive, but also takes the future child's health/welfare into account, as it is of proven benefit in reducing the risk of HIV to the offspring.

Legal parental responsibility, enshrined in UK law[7], starts from the moment that the child is born alive, and lasts until adulthood (18 years), but, ethically, prospective parents' responsibility starts with the conception project. Explicit in some legislation (UK), the principle of child welfare is arguably implicit in other countries. For instance, in France, it is still forbidden to help single women or women in a lesbian couple to conceive, or to offer posthumous treatment, and, 'in case of a conflict (between the couple requesting treatment and the physician and his/her team), this usually means the intervention of a psychologist, referral to an ethics committee, or recourse to legal procedure'[1]. In countries which, like France, have a legal system inspired by Roman law[8], the legal procedure is common; thus, a judge must authorize both recipient and donor couples in the case of embryo donation ('accueil', i.e. 'welcome'). There are indeed numerous variations in the law allowing access to assisted reproductive technologies (ART) in European countries[9], with many requiring marriage or a couple to live together for a while, symbols of different visions of the family, and of society. Such requirements translated into professional codes, or legal norms, are implicit in consideration of the welfare of the child.

Apart from the social context, physicians will often consider it their duty to warn and assist (or not) persons at high risk of transmitting disease, whether it be viral (such as HIV or hepatitis) or genetic, and will in this difficult equation consider not only the health of the woman who may be endangered by a pregnancy, but also that of the offspring.

Thus, the welfare of the child has at least two components: physical (or medical) and psychosocial. In this chapter, we first discuss the medical factors and refer the reader to chapters in this or our previous volume[10], where detailed analysis is made of several known physical risks to the offspring of ART. It must, of course, be stated that the welfare of the future child is also taken into account in the usual context of planning for a healthy pregnancy which does not need to be assisted by technology, by advising women on taking folic acid and controlling their weight and alcohol intake, and providing a safe pregnancy by means of good antenatal and delivery care (which leaves the African continent very bereft, with its high incidence of maternal death, and fistulas due to poor delivery care, followed by social exclusion of the mother and the inevitable consequences for the welfare of her child). Many of these decisions are taken at national level and are in the realm of public-health policy.

The second part is without doubt more complex to justify, as psychosocial decisions to 'screen', advise or even discourage women or couples from undertaking a pregnancy are not taken lightly in the modern context of respecting liberty and 'procreative autonomy'. If we assume, along with J. S. Mill, that the sole reason for the state to interfere in the lives of individuals is that their behavior may harm others, then it is possible to argue that we are currently over-regulated in the area of the provision of assisted reproduction[11]. End-points are more difficult to measure for physicians and scientists who need to be aware of findings in social sciences and anthropology, as to the effect on the child of single motherhood, for instance, but recent studies have certainly helped professionals to make decisions based on evidence rather than prejudice. An obvious extreme example of denying women their reproductive autonomy is the well-known enforced sterilization of the mentally disabled which happened in the USA, Sweden, the UK and other countries. In the UK a judge decided that all similar cases should be reviewed by tribunal, before permission is granted[12].

We also need to examine the standards and implementation of a policy to take into account the welfare of the child. Such assessment and measure of the 'welfare principle'[4] range from maximum to minimum standard with either very strict or very loose criteria: a 'reasonable' approach is generally agreed to be sensible.

Finally, there will be cases where prospective/intended parents and the medical team will disagree as to whether any treatment is appropriate or not. We also need to examine solutions to this problem.

MEDICAL ASPECTS OF ART AND WELFARE CONSIDERATIONS

This aspect of the concept of welfare of the child is arguably easier to assess, as it deals with outcomes, which in many cases have been subjected to analysis in large numbers, and enters the realm of evidence-based findings. It may involve the complications of ART, or the risks of transmissible disease (viral or genetic). The former would apply to all patients, and be related to the technique used; the latter applies to some patients whose condition entails an inherent and personal extra risk.

When the evidence becomes strong that a technique[13] leads to a high incidence of complications, the onus is on the profession to inform our patients, and use good practice to reduce complications or do without the technique: this applies to subjects discussed in other chapters of this book or the previous volume[10], which are only briefly mentioned here. Amongst the direct risks of ART, that of iatrogenic multiple pregnancy is the most important and well known[14–16]. This means that single embryo transfer should be considered more and more in ideal circumstances[17]. There are also known or unknown consequences of new technologies, sometimes described as progress before there is such evidence, for instance, intracytoplasmic sperm injection (ICSI), with the use of testicular sperm is not allowed in The Netherlands on the grounds of safety.

Other risks not directly related to the techniques of ART are those relating to HIV-positive parent(s) asking for help to conceive and also diminish the risk of transmission to offspring, or to parents with a high genetic risk or risk of trans-mitting a serious disease requesting preimplantation genetic diagnosis (PGD)[18].

One of the questions arising here[1] is: 'in what physical (and social) conditions is it acceptable to bring a child into the world?' It is important to note that the legal term used in the UK differentiates between the future child, whose 'welfare' must be taken into account, and the 'best interest' of a born child, which is considered to be paramount[7]. This terminology is both legally and symbolically important.

Giving information to the prospective parents is key to their autonomy, to allow them to 'consent' or indeed dissent to what is proposed, and understand the risks, if present. Difficulties in explaining risk, and its two components, incidence and gravity, must not be underestimated; although it is relatively easy to understand the meaning of a 90% risk of malformation in a case of early rubella, it is more dif-ficult to integrate a risk of 4–5% in a case of toxoplasmosis, where prospective parents may prefer to interrupt a pregnancy, although the fetus has a 95% chance to be normal. The gravity of the future child's possible impairment is another aspect to consider, and may be subjectively assessed; for instance, in an experi-ment of (directive?) information and counseling[19], some prospective parents choose not to terminate the pregnancy after an ultrasound diagnosis of limb abnormalities followed by a visit to a specialist center looking after infants affect-ed by similar malformations.

This means that the medical profession has to be open-minded and avoid paternalistic attitudes, in order to respect parental autonomy. Particularly difficult is the taking into consideration of the expected 'quality of life' of the future child. The criteria allowing one to determine whether a given life is worth accepting are very personal, and may vary tremendously for different future parents and even for the same prospective parents with time. Rare are the cases where the estimated future quality of life, one determinant of the welfare of the future child, can be determined with certainty, but we can refer to court decisions to enlighten the argument. In a famous French case[20], a pregnant woman affected by rubella was told that she was clear, by mistake. After the birth of a severely affected child with deafness, partial blindness and cardiac malformation, she argued in court that she would have requested a termination of pregnancy had she been fully informed. The legal arguments were fierce, and it was argued that it was preferable for the child to exist, although severely handicapped, than be unborn; the Cassation Court (appeal of the appeal) decided to condemn the practitioner to offer compensation for the child's suffering and the cost of special care. Nevertheless, this has since been superseded[21]: similar cases in the future would be compensated by the national insurance system.

But whatever the difficulties of assessing risks we know about, it is imperative also to follow children born by means of ART, as some studies show a small increased risk depending on the method of treatment used[22], although this may be due to the primary condition of subfertility of the parents. Only this will enable us to inform our patients better so that we can enable them to make an informed decision whether to have treatment (or not).

PSYCHOSOCIAL ASPECTS OF THE WELFARE-OF-THE-CHILD PRINCIPLE

Physicians are generally not trained in psychology or social sciences, and thus need access to a team of experts for consultation, in order to appraise relevant welfare-of-the-child factors in these fields. Several social components have been studied in the general and subfertile populations, especially family structure, and knowledge of one's origins. The former has seen many changes in the past two generations, with an increasing number of children being looked after in divorced or 'second' families, by same-sex parents or by single mothers. The legally enshrined provision (or lack) of ART in such cases varies amongst countries, as 'providing assisted conception in these circumstances recognizes as legitimate the wish for descendants of those who refuse marriage, partnership or heterosexuality as a way of life and as the only suitable framework for raising children'[1].

First, with regard to family structure, French ART law explicitly views widowhood and single women as less than acceptable planned circumstances for the future child. The ethical and legal issues concerning posthumous conception with cryopreserved sperm are studied elsewhere in detail in this volume (see Chapter 3). But perhaps even more tragic is the case whereby cryopreserved embryos cannot be transferred after the death of the husband, thus interrupting the 'parental project' objectified by the fact that embryos have been created *in vitro*, without consideration for the wish of the prospective and widowed mother. The case of Mrs Pires[23] is probably the best example of the deleterious consequences of ideological legal concepts with the only options of destruction or gift to another couple, by two successive ART laws in 1994[24] and 2004[25]. In similar circumstances, pragmatic options can be codified, whilst taking into account the welfare of the child[26].

French legislation has given the same dogmatic refusal to treat same sex-couples or single women, a debate where prejudice may be replaced by evidence now that several studies have shown very few measurable differences from the donor offspring of heterosexual couples[27]. As for surrogacy, which could be argued not to threaten the family structure of the intending parents[28] (European Society of Human Reproduction and Embryology (ESHRE) Taskforce 10), measures may be taken to avoid exploitation of the vulnerable carrying mother, with its possible consequences for the informed future child[29]. Family structure and the knowledge of one's origins inter-relate from some aspects. Certainly, when donor insemination is used for single women or lesbian couples, several studies have already shown that information is more readily given to offspring than it is in heterosexual couples where a psychosocial (and legal) father is present. We know from the adoption model that it is better to tell adopted children the truth about their origins; indeed, it has been argued that 'untold facts' or secrets have deleterious consequences on the psychology of the child, including lack of trust towards their parents, especially if the secret is disclosed in an uncontrolled manner to the offspring. When ART uses the gametes of the 'social' parents, there is no reason to think that it should affect the welfare of the future child, but when gametes are donated, it may still be difficult for prospective parents to accept without reluctance their duty to inform the offspring, especially those who go against their social or religious traditions in order to have a child of their own. Indeed and furthermore, the well-known difference between secrecy and lack of anonymity of gamete donors has been the subject of intense debates, especially with regard to the future offspring's 'right to know'. The interest of the future child concerning the matter of access to the identity of the genetic/donor gamete provider(s) is of particular complexity, and despite the positions of very active lobbies, and the unconvincing[30] arguments in the realm of human rights, it cannot be said that the matter is definitely settled. Reference, in this respect, is frequently made to Art. 7 of the United Nations Convention about the rights of children[31] 'to know their parents and to be cared by them, as far as possible'. It may be argued that this statement does not necessarily mean the right to know their 'genetic parents', but rather the initial intending parents; in fact this frequently misquoted phrase refers to specific historical conditions, and the tragic situation of South American children born during political turmoil, who were forcedly abducted from their parents, and often adopted by people linked to the very same dictatorship responsible for their parents' death.

It is also interesting to note that the difference in attitude with regard to anonymity of gamete donors reflects a difference in the family structure in Europe, with more acknowledgment of the reality of the biological process in Anglo-Saxon and Scandinavian countries, and emphasis on the 'social' definition and role of the family in other European continental countries. However, one may wonder why the 'double-track policy' (i.e. the choice offered to donors to be anonymous or not, and similarly the choice offered to the couple to obtain anonymous or non-anonymous donation), once accepted in several countries such as The Netherlands, has now been abandoned, and not even considered in France, still strongly attached to the principle of anonymity. In both cases, preference seems to stem from ideology rather than pragmatic evaluation of the diverse attitudes, a caveat for any diktat concerning blanket-rule for the welfare of the future child, when there is no evidence of harm[27]. The compromise opinion still favors parental choice in view of the lack of evidence one way or the other[32].

Finally, the analogy with the case of adopted children born 'under X', a system which prevails in a minority of countries such as France and Luxemburg, is a useful reference. This process, where there is no mother's name on the birth certificate, was created in order to protect the interests, the wishes and sometimes the life of the biological mother, and may conflict with the desire of the child to know of his/her origin when informed about the procedure which has led to the adoption. It has recently been subjected to the wisdom of the European Court of

Human Rights[33]. The Court stated that the principle of subsidiarity was to be applied in the case, respecting national laws, which in the UK would mean that a child's best interest is paramount. Recent disputes in France have finally led to a subtle legislative change, with creation of an agency charged to collect all the requests of offspring after the age of 18 and adopted from unknown parents (including women delivered under X), and to attempt to trace the identity of the delivering mother by matching dates in registries of maternity units. The ultimate goal is to contact the delivering mother, and to ask her whether she wishes to have news of and eventually direct contact with her child. This example reminds us that the welfare of the child has an important bearing on the welfare of the offspring who needs not be legally a child any longer, and also underlines gender inequality: the father has only 2 months to find a putative child, and to start the legal procedure to 'recognize' the infant and put his name on the birth certificate.

Finally, other possible psychosocial risks are in the realm of danger of neglect or abuse. Neglect may stem from parental inability to care through physical or mental disablement[34], domestic violence or drug and alcohol abuse. There is no doubt that in such cases a multidisciplinary approach is necessary, in order to assess the risk to the welfare of the child. The complexity of assessing the degree of harm is discussed below.

ASSESSING THE WELFARE OF THE CHILD AND IMPLEMENTING POLICIES: THREE LEVELS, THREE APPROACHES

The criteria for measuring the welfare of the child range from minimal standard to maximal[4]. The strictest is the 'maximal welfare' standard, a high standard where no medical assistance to conceive should be provided when there are indications that the life conditions of the future child will not be optimal. At the opposite end of the spectrum lies the 'minimal welfare' standard, where medical assistance to reproduction is only unacceptable if there is a risk of serious harm, or the life quality of the future child is so low that it would have been better off being unborn, a statement rarely made, even in courts of law. The middle standard is that of 'reasonable welfare': assistance is acceptable if the future person will have the ability and opportunities to realize those dimensions and goals that in general make a human life valuable.

Thus, in correlation, one can evolve three degrees/levels of participation for the ART team. The first degree is non-participation, when the predicted level of well-being of the future child is estimated to fall below a minimal threshold (e.g. when there is a high risk of serious harm); the physician should not participate in the project, and indeed might be morally obligated to refuse participation in order to protect a future child. This may mean that the couple or person is referred to another agent for help with regard to the problems detected, and that they may move a step above the minimal threshold after resolution.

From that minimal threshold, and up to the level of reasonable well-being, the physician may participate, but collaboration is not obligatory; this is the degree/level of possible participation. From the level of reasonable well-being and above, the physician should assist but can be excused on the basis of conscientious objections, when it becomes a duty to pass on the care to another physician; this level is participation (direct or by proxy if referral is made).

Thus, decision-making may comprise three approaches: refusal, acceptance of a patient (couple/single woman) or acceptance with conditions. The last may apply at a level between the minimal and reasonable threshold standards, for instance where a prospective parent is asked to ensure withdrawal from addictive drugs before fertility treatment is offered, which would, when achieved, lead to a more 'reasonable' level, and certainly above the minimal threshold. As is often the case, circumstances may vary tremendously between apparently similar cases, and it is essential to have a pluridisciplinary team approach, which includes psychological assessment.

Refusal of treatment may be because the welfare of the child falls below the minimal threshold standard, or because the practitioner has a conscientious objection to particular treatments. In the latter case, there should be alternative sources of treatment indicated to the patient(s), but when ART is refused for a 'high risk of serious harm' (two addicted parents for instance, or both totally unable to care for a child for other reasons), all attempts must be made to seek multidisciplinary advice and counseling, with full explanation given to the couple. Conditional treatment may be offered if objective evidence is present of changes likely to bring the welfare of the child above the minimal threshold.

The process/procedure for assessment that needs to be used is another problematic area[35]. The main point is whether all intending parents requiring ART should have an assessment, or only those where the welfare of the child is assessed to be of minimal standard or between minimal and intermediate. Until November 2005, the Human Fertilisation and Embryology Authority (HFEA) guidance in the Code of Practice[36] advised clinics to write to all general practitioners (GPs) of patients seeking licensed treatments in the UK. After the results of a public consultation document, new guidance has been issued by the HFEA at the end of 2005[37], stating that 'there should be a presumption to provide treatment, unless there is evidence that the child to be born, or any existing child of the family, is likely to suffer serious medical, physical or psychological harm', and that 'medical and social information will now be collected from the patients themselves, with follow up to GPs or other agencies only when clinics judge there to be a risk of serious harm'. This latest guidance is similar in spirit to the 'three levels, three approaches' described above, and also fits with a recent parliamentary commission report[3], which overtly states that the clinician in charge may be trusted to make the right decision. The only drawback of this position is that it may herald a danger of return to the paternalism of old. In cases of concern, the HFEA still recommends contacting the GP, who has in the UK a privileged position of being the provider of core services and the referral agent, thus making him/her well placed to be a co-agent with the ART team in decision-making. Different agencies, psychological, social and medical, as well as patient support groups in the case of serious disease, may be consulted, but it is probably best to enlist such agencies in selected cases rather than in all cases of ART.

CONCLUSION

Taking into account the welfare of the child stems from the responsible practice of fertility specialists. There are different kinds of risks for the future child, those linked to the safety of ART, and those linked to the particular circumstances of the woman or couple undergoing treatment. Very risky procedures are an extreme example which prejudice both the welfare of the child and the present and future respect of the specialty (such as reproductive cloning, or formation of hybrids). These procedures cannot always be controlled by law, national or international; proper appraisal of research is mainly in the hands of the medical and scientific professions, all sharing responsibility.

It is essential that taking into account the welfare of the child should be achieved without prejudice, or a priori concepts and/or religious beliefs. Thus, policies that are enshrined in codes of practice and fully transparent to the public are probably better and fairer than the casuistic appraisal of the clinical team in charge of treatment, although, after following general guidelines, national and international, some casuistry is inevitable. Opinions and society are in constant change, and we must take into consideration the opinion of society as a whole, including those most directly concerned. Informed decision-making after multi-disciplinary exchanges (with participation of the future parents, members of the medical team and psychologists, ethicists, sociologists, etc.), as in the field of 'clinical ethics', leads to a more a subtle, pragmatic, non-directive approach. Furthermore, international professional societies and their ethics deliberations[38] may serve as reference to further analysis of national policies sometimes based on tradition and prejudice rather than evidence.

Finally, in a broad sense, it may be argued that embryo research is a field which is related to the welfare of future children in ART, particularly when it aims to improve the quality and efficiency of treatment, and prevent anomalies. For instance, the newly formed French Agence de la biomédecine will evaluate medical and biological activities, including the consequences of ART for both users of the techniques and the ensuing children, and set up a system of surveillance of all techniques[25].

Indeed, follow-up of children born from our assistance is necessary in order to gather evidence on possible complications of ART. This is certainly an endeavor which can be international, based on the model of European *in vitro* fertilization (IVF) monitoring[39] and other databases that give reliable information regarding large numbers, and is more likely to proceed and succeed than fantasies of international regulations. We may also challenge the materialistic notion of caveat emptor sometimes used in libertarian societies who regard patients buying health care as if they were buying any other goods; a caring society should offer a degree of protection to its members, and even more to the future vulnerable party, the hoped-for child of our patients.

REFERENCES

1. Bateman S. When reproductive freedom encounters medical responsibility: changing conceptions of reproductive choice. In Current Practice and Controversies in Assisted Reproduction. Report of a meeting on 'Medical, Social and Ethical Aspects of Assisted Reproduction'. Geneva: WHO, 2002.
2. Human Fertilisation and Embryology Act 1990. London: HMSO, 1990.
3. House of Commons. Human Reproductive Technologies and the Law. London: HMSO, 2005.
4. Pennings G. Measuring the welfare of the child: in search of the appropriate evaluation principle. Hum Reprod 1999; 14: 1146–50.
5. de Wert G, Berghmans R. In vitro fertilisation: access, responsibility of the doctor and welfare of the child. In Dooley D, Dalla-Vorgia P, Garanis-Papadatos T, McCarthy J, eds. The Ethics of New Reproductive Technologies. Cases and Questions. New York: Berghahn Books, 2003: 154–8.
6. Paton vs. UK (1990) 3 EHHRR 408.
7. Children Act 1989. London: HMSO, 1989.
8. Dickens BM. Interfaces of assisted reproduction ethics and law. In Shenfield F, Sureau C, eds. Ethical Dilemmas in Assisted Reproduction. Carnforth, UK: Parthenon Publishing, 1997: 77–81.
9. IFFS Surveillance 04. Fertil Steril 2004; 81 (Suppl 4).
10. Shenfield F, Sureau C, eds. Ethical dilemmas in Reproduction. New York: Parthenon Publishing, 2002.
11. McLean S. Testimony to the House of Commons. Human Reproductive Technologies and the Law. London: HMSO, 2005.
12. Kennedy I, Grubb A. Medical Law: Text with Materials, 2nd edn. London: Butterworths, 1994: 718–29.
13. Ombelet W, Cadron I, Gerris J, et al. Obstetric and perinatal outcome of 1655 ICSI and 3974 IVF singleton and 1102 ICSI and 2901 IVF twin births: a comparative analysis. Reprod Biomed Online 2005; 11: 76–85.
14. Shenfield F. The responsibility of the fertility specialist in preventing multiple pregnancies in ART. Reprod Biomed Online 2003; 7 (Suppl 2): 526–7.
15. ESHRE Taskforce on Ethics and Law 6. Ethical issues related to multiple pregnancies in medically assisted reproduction. Hum Reprod 2003; 18: 1976–9.
16. Cohen J. Multiple pregnancies and our responsibility to ART children. In Shenfield F, Sureau C, eds. Ethical Dilemmas in Reproduction. New York: Parthenon Publishing, 2002.
17. Gerris J, De Sutter P, de Neuburg D, et al. A real life prospective health economics study of elective single embryo transfer versus two embryo transfer in first IVF/ICSI cycles. Hum Reprod 2004; 19: 917–23.

18. ESHRE Ethics and Law Taskforce 5. Preimplantation genetic diagnosis. Hum Reprod 2003; 18: 649–51.

19. Boulot B, Devanz ML. Prise en charge psychologique a l'annonce d'une malformation. Oral communication, 8th National Day for French Fetal Medicine Society, 1996.

20. TGI 13 January 1992 Appeal 17 December 1993 and 17 November 2000, Arrêt Perruche, Cassation 17 November 2000.

21. Loi no 2002-303 du 4 mars 2002, relative aux droits des maladies et à la qualité du système de santé (JORF 5/3/02).

22. Bonduelle M, Wennerholm UB, Loft A, et al. A multi-centre cohort study of the physical health of 5-year-old children conceived after intracytoplasmic sperm injection, in vitro fertilization and natural conception. Hum Reprod, 2004; 20: 413–19.

23. Arrêt 59 P, 1ère chambre, Cour de cassation 9 janvier 1996 (Pires).

24. Loi no 94-653 du 29 juillet 1994, relative au respect du corps humain.

25. Loi no 2004-800 du 6 août 2004 relative à la bioéthique.

26. ESHRE Law and Ethics Taskforce II. The cryopreservation of human embryos. Hum Reprod 2001; 16: 1049–50.

27. Golombok S, Mac Cullum F, Goodman E, Rutter M. Families with children conceived by DI: a follow up at age 12. Child Dev 2002; 73: 952–68.

28. ESHRE Taskforce on Ethics and Law 10. Surrogacy. Hum Reprod 2005; 20: 2705–7.

29. English V, Sommerville A, Brinsden PF. Surrogacy. In Shenfield F, Sureau C, eds. Ethical Dilemmas in Assisted Reproduction. Carnforth, UK: Parthenon Publishing, 1997: 35–7.

30. Shenfield F. To know or not to know the identity of one's genetic parent(s): a question of human rights? In Healy DL, Kovacs GT, McLachlan R, Rodriguez-Armas O, eds. IFFS 2001: Reproductive Medicine in the Twenty-first Century. London, UK: Parthenon Publishing, 2002: 78–85.

31. United Nations Convention on the Rights of the Child 1989, ART. 7, adopted 20 November 1989.

32. ESHRE Taskforce on Ethics and Law III. Gamete and embryo donation. Hum Reprod 2002; 17: 1407–8.

33. Strasbourg European Court of Human Rights req no42 326/98. Mme Odièvre vs. France, 133/2/2003.

34. De Wert G. ESHRE joint pre-congress course on Ethics and Law and Psychology and Counseling, Annual Meeting, Copenhagen, 2005.

35. HFEA Consultation Document on the Welfare of the Child. www.hfea.gov.uk. Accessed 2005.

36. HFEA Code of Practice. www.hfea.gov.uk. Accessed 2005.

37. HFEA, New Guidance on Welfare of the Child Assessment, CH (05) 04, 2/11/2005.

38. ASRM Ethics Committee. Child-rearing ability and the provision of fertility services: The Ethics Committee of the American Society for Reproductive Medicine. Fertil Steril 2004; 82: 564–7.

39. Andersen AN, Gianaroli L, Felberbaum R, et al. The European IVF-monitoring programme (EIM), European Society of Human Reproduction and Embryology (ESHRE). Assisted reproductive technology in Europe, 2001. Results generated from European registers by ESHRE. Hum Reprod 2005; 20: 1158–76.

Chapter 7

Preimplantation genetic diagnosis for hereditary disorders that do not show a simple Mendelian pattern: an ethical exploration

Guido de Wert and Joep P M Geraedts

INTRODUCTION

In order to define the topic of this chapter, a few terms need to be clarified: first, the term *preimplantation genetic diagnosis* (PGD). PGD is generally defined as testing embryos or oocytes for Mendelian and chromosomal defects. In view of this definition, PGD for hereditary disorders that do not show a simple Mendelian pattern might be a *contradiction in terms*. Clearly, we need a more 'inclusive' definition of PGD, which does not a priori exclude more complex patterns of inheritance.

Second, the different patterns of inheritance should be defined more precisely. In principle, five simple modes can be distinguished: autosomal dominant, autosomal recessive, X-linked recessive, X-linked dominant and Y-linked. In practice, only the first three are relevant. Besides these modes of nuclear inheritance, mitochondrial inheritance also exists. It shows completely maternal inheritance. From this, it might not be concluded that all diseases which, when studying the pedigree, seem to follow a more complex pattern cannot result from simple point mutations in individual genes. The first level of complexity results from incomplete penetrance and variable expression. Incomplete penetrance means that a number of genotypically affected carriers do not demonstrate any symptoms of the condition at all. Variable expression means that not all disease carriers show the same severity of the condition, and suggests that environmental factors are involved. Furthermore, pleiotropy is known as the situation in which one and the same mutation can cause more than one effect. The breast cancer mutations BRCA-1 and -2 are good examples of this. They can either have no effect at all (non-penetrance) or result in breast cancer on the one hand or ovarian cancer on the other. In recent literature, the term *complex* disorders is preferred for all genetic conditions that are not strictly Mendelian or chromosomal in nature.

Complex disorders might result from two or more genes (polygenic inheritance) as well as from more than one gene in combination with environmental factors. The latter situation is sometimes called multifactorial inheritance. If more than one gene is involved, sometimes a distinction is made between major and minor genes. The major gene has a profound phenotypic effect, whereas the minor gene(s) can be regarded as modifiers(s) of the phenotypic expression. In this chapter, we consider all disorders that are not caused by mutations in one gene with *complete* penetrance as hereditary disorders that do not show a simple Mendelian pattern.

Third, we refer to the term *disorders*. Acknowledging the conceptual difficulties regarding the concept of 'disease' and the related inter- and intracultural differences, this chapter does not comment on PGD for predispositions for complex *normal* characteristics – it is confined to the so-called 'medical model'[1,2].

The ethics of PGD *as such* is beyond the scope of this chapter. It is simply presumed that both *in vitro* fertilization/intracytoplasmic sperm injection (IVF/ICSI) and PGD can be morally justified, and that the deontological and consequentialist arguments in favor of prohibiting (post-conception) PGD (e.g. Germany, Italy) are not convincing – or even bizarre[2–6]. The ethical question, then, runs as follows: can PGD for disorders that do not follow simple inheritance patterns be morally justified, and if so, on what conditions?

ETHICAL EXPLORATION

Preimplantation susceptibility testing: 'pros and cons'

Most authors and committees who have discussed the issue of prenatal testing and/or PGD for disorders that do not follow a simple Mendelian inheritance pattern are highly reluctant about, if not completely opposed to, this type of testing. The American Institute of Medicine's (IOM) 'Committee on Assessing Genetic Risks', for instance, recommended in its section on predictive testing for *late-onset* disorders that, in the current state of knowledge, reproductive interventions, including prenatal diagnosis (and, we assume, PGD), should not be conducted for determining increased genetic susceptibility to multifactorial disorders[7]. Unfortunately, the report did not make clear how new knowledge could potentially influence this provisional negative point of view, nor whether the IOM's Committee would consider prenatal and/or preimplantation testing for more complex *early*-onset disorders to be acceptable.

The guidance provided by the Canadian Royal Commission on New Reproductive Technologies is even more restrictive: doctors should not offer prenatal susceptibility testing, as this type of testing is unable to provide useful and relevant information ('having a susceptibility gene does not necessarily mean developing the disorder'), the incidence of the disorder is affected by complex but potentially controllable environmental factors, and the disorders concerned do not develop until adulthood[8]. Furthermore, the Commission stresses that, like prenatal testing for late-onset *dominant* disorders, prenatal susceptibility testing puts children in a very vulnerable situation if they are shown to be at higher risk; such testing may well imply potential harm to the self-image and the potential for stigmatization and discrimination. And finally, so the Commission argues, since everyone carries an unknown number of susceptibility genes, there is no way to ensure that children are free of all genetic susceptibilities – in fact it is unlikely that any of us are. We may safely presume that, according to this Committee, the same objections would apply to *preimplantation* susceptibility testing.

Some philosophers, however, argue that (prenatal and) preimplantation susceptibility testing should be provided. Carson Strong's view draws upon the dominant conception of the role of the physician: the purpose of reproductive genetic counseling is to help prospective parents dealing with disease, including susceptibilities for disease, to have healthy children. As long as requests for prenatal/ preimplantation susceptibility testing are within this domain (the 'medical model'), physicians should strive to be *non-directive*[6]. Discussing the ethics of prenatal testing and selective abortion, Steinbock argues that the principle of reproductive freedom is of paramount importance. This means 'that women have the right to choose to abort even if they choose for reasons that most people consider trivial or frivolous. . . . Physicians . . . should ultimately respect the woman's right to make this decision and her related right to have information that she deems relevant to the decision'[9]. A separate question is whether a specific test should be made 'generally available'. Steinbock concludes that while the doctor may, or even should, discuss his hesitations and concerns regarding 'bizarre' susceptibility tests with the client, ultimately the decision should rest with the client – *assuming that she is willing to pay for it*. We presume, that, according to Steinbock, the same logic would apply to *PGD* for susceptibilities. In a more recent publication, she states that while it would not make sense to undergo IVF and PGD in order to avoid the birth of a child at higher risk of developing (for example) multifactorial, late-onset, Alzheimer's disease (AD) – which typically develops in the 70s, 80s or even 90s – if a couple were already undergoing IVF for infertility, and were particularly concerned about (this type of) AD, they might want to use PGD to reduce the risk[2]. What should one think of these views?

While the American and Canadian Committees rightly point to some of the problems of prenatal/preimplantation testing for increased genetic susceptibility, their seemingly *categorical* rejection of this type of testing is a *non sequitur*. The Canadian Committee's arguments are especially weak; after all:

(1) One cannot reasonably argue that only reproductive tests which provide 100% certainty are useful;

(2) Relevant environmental factors are often not known and/or not controllable;

(3) The suggestion that all multifactorial disorders are, *per se*, *late-onset* disorders is simply wrong (see 'Cases' below);

(4) Potential harm to the self-image of future children prenatally identified as carriers of genetic susceptibilities are to be avoided if such testing were to take place for selective purposes;

(5)   While trying to conceive children *completely free* from genetic susceptibilities for diseases is clearly a misguided effort, is does not necessarily follow that prenatal testing for a specific, highly penetrant predisposition is unwarranted in each and every case.

Strong and, in particular, Steinbock, fail to present a proper balance between respect for clients' procreative autonomy on the one hand and professional responsibility on the other. Strong's suggestion that the traditional ideal of non-directiveness obliges the physician to give *unconditional* support to his clients, whatever they request, is simplistic. After all, a medical doctor is not a marionette. Steinbock does not convincingly argue that procreative freedom includes the (apparently unqualified) right to have *all* the information that prospective parents deem relevant for making reproductive decisions. To argue that doctors should ultimately comply even with 'bizarre' requests for susceptibility testing, on the condition that clients pay for it, de facto makes a mockery of medical ethics.

We conclude, then, that while the American and Canadian Committees mentioned are too restrictive, the philosophers mentioned are too permissive. Good clinical practice requires some sort of a 'middle of the road' approach.

Relevant variables

The questions 'Which prenatal/preimplantation genetic tests should be performed?' and 'Where precisely to draw the line?' are notably difficult to answer. A number of relevant variables should be considered *simultaneously*. Some of these are more or less 'traditional', including:

(1)   The disorder's severity, taking into account its variable expression and the availability of treatment options;

(2)   The age of onset of the disease; *and*

(3)   The penetrance of the genetic defect, i.e. the probability that the genotype will be reflected in the phenotype and will have consequences for health[1,10,11].

The case for (prenatal and) preimplantation genetic testing is strongest where the disorder/handicap is severe, preventive and/or therapeutic interventions are not available, the disorder has an early-onset and the penetrance of the genetic defect is complete – and *vice versa*. Before considering whether there are any additional variables to be taken into account, we first briefly comment on the last of these 'traditional' variables.

PGD for *low*-penetrance predispositions may be questioned for several reasons and from various perspectives. Whether or not one accepts all or some of these arguments depends, of course, on one's view on the relevant background theories. First, from a so-called 'fetalist' perspective, one might argue that a decision not to transfer embryos carrying only a predisposition is at odds with the status of the (preimplantation) embryo; a low-penetrance mutation/polymorphism may not provide a sufficiently weighty reason to justify embryo selection. Some people might claim that this problem could be avoided by a *sequential first and second polar body biopsy*, as this would amount to the testing of *oocytes* , i.e. *preconception* PGD. This, however, seems to be a highly debatable classification. Clearly, people who think that the preimplantation embryo has no independent moral status or that only very limited respect should be accorded to preimplantation embryos may not support this first argument. A second argument is that IVF/PGD for low-penetrance mutations would be disproportionate, given the potential health risks and burdens of IVF/ICSI. Insofar as these health risks concern the health of *women* undergoing IVF/ICSI, this argument is paternalistic. People may differ as to whether paternalism is justified or not – depending on their position regarding patient autonomy. An absolute antipaternalist might argue that it is up to the prospective parents themselves to balance the pros and cons, after being adequately informed. Some proponents of this second objection might focus on the possible health risks of the biopsy for *progeny*; even though findings of follow-up studies so far seem to be reassuring, the picture is not yet completely clear. We would suggest that clients' autonomy has its limits; below a certain penetrance, the risk/burdens of IVF should be considered out of proportion. No doubt, any threshold is always to some extent arbitrary. To conclude, however, that, because any threshold is to some degree arbitrary, a threshold should be rejected altogether, simply is a non sequitur.

A third argument concerns the just allocation of scarce resources, both in terms of finances *and* in terms of personnel. The core of a just health-care system is universal access to an adequate level of health care. The perennial question is: what should be counted as an adequate level/decent minimum of health care? We would argue that collective funding of IVF/PGD for susceptibilities irrespective of their penetrance would be difficult to justify. The 'argument from justice' does not become irrelevant if preimplantation susceptibility testing were not to be reimbursed[12]. After all, performing such tests may well have detrimental effects for clinical practice in view of the labor-intensiveness of, for instance, developing mutation-specific assays. The postponement of IVF/PGD cycles for couples truly *at high risk* would be morally problematic. All other things being equal, IVF/PGD centers should give priority to PGD for 'high(er)-penetrance' mutations.

But where, then, should one draw the line between low- and high-penetrance mutations? Some people will argue that the penetrance should be close to 100% (i.e. almost complete) in order to qualify for preimplantation testing. This view seems to be far too restrictive, and is at odds with current clinical practice. After all, there is a strong consensus that PGD for medical sex selection, preventing the birth of boys suffering from X-linked disorders, is justified – even though the risk for male embryos/future boys is 'just' 50%. In view of this, the issue becomes whether the penetrance of predispositions should be at least 50% in order to qualify for PGD, or whether a (somewhat) lower penetrance could be acceptable as well – at least in the case of *severe, early-onset* disorders.

Apart from the penetrance of the specific mutation, the severity of the disorder and its age of onset, at least two additional aspects need to be taken into account when weighing the pros and cons of PGD for disorders that do not follow simple inheritance patterns. First, in some cases, *primary prevention* may be possible, for instance by modifying the relevant environmental factors, with the aim of avoiding exposure to those factors that trigger the disease, or by medical interventions. Obviously, if the disorder could be prevented altogether by simply avoiding specific food or taking particular drugs or vitamins, it would make little sense to opt for IVF/embryo selection. Second, in some cases (e.g. testing for polygenic disorders, where other genes than those tested for or environmental factors are involved), there may be *residual* genetic risks after PGD for the major gene; as a general rule, the higher is the residual risk, the less proportionate would be the IVF/preimplantation susceptibility testing). Significant residual risks may be problematic for various reasons (from different perspectives). To begin with, it may well turn out that the concerns and worries of prospective parents regarding the health of their future child will not be alleviated by PGD; embryo selection may not bring 'reproductive confidence'. Furthermore, residual risks may be problematic in view of the doctor's responsibility to take into account the health interests of future children conceived by assisted reproductive technologies (ART). Obviously, the harm-probability ratio will be important for handling these situations. In any case, high risks of serious harm should be avoided.

It has been suggested that we take into account another (third) additional variable: we should discern the case of people who undergo IVF/ICSI just in order to perform PGD for a specific susceptibility, on the one hand, and the case of couples who apply for this type of PGD in the context of IVF for infertility, on the other hand[2,13]. One might argue that in the latter case, testing for a *lower*-penetrance mutation could be justified. After all, these people will opt for IVF anyway; the risks/burdens of this procedure are proportionate and justified because it is the only way for them to reproduce. The difference between these types of situation seems, however, to be only gradual, as one may have to start additional IVF/ICSI cycles as a consequence of the selection of embryos.

Cases

The complexity of the issues at hand becomes even clearer when looking at some cases for which the request of PGD might be envisaged. The current exploration serves to illustrate both that we need to develop *differentiated* guidelines regarding PGD for disorders with inheritance patterns that do not strictly follow the Mendelian rules, and that it will be rather difficult to reach consensus regarding each individual case. The cases presented follow chronological order.

Congenital malformations

Holoprosencephaly (HPE) HPE is a developmental anomaly of the forebrain and mid-face. Familial cases, with a pattern of autosomal dominant inheritance, are not rare. There is a great clinical variability within families, ranging from (alobar

HPE and) cyclopia to normal phenotype. According to Verlinsky *et al.*, PGD/selective transfer may be a more attractive option for couples at risk of having a child with familiar HPE than regular prenatal diagnosis/selective termination of pregnancy, because almost one-third of carriers of relevant sonic hedgehog (SHH) mutations may be clinically unaffected[14]. In view of the severity of symptoms in the majority of the cases, and the high penetrance of the relevant mutations, PGD seems to be justified from a moral point of view.

Of course, clients need to be informed that prenatal ultrasound would be more informative than PGD. In this respect it is important to know that the earliest age at diagnosis was at 15 weeks' pregnancy, and the mean menstrual age at prenatal diagnosis was 24.7 and 24.8 weeks, in two of the larger series[15,16]. For selective pregnancy termination this is rather late in pregnancy; in many countries, a third-trimester termination is illegal. Irrespective of this regulatory aspect, we assume that many couples would favor PGD above prenatal diagnosis for this reason. However, these series consisted of sporadic cases of holoprosencephaly. It is likely that the diagnosis of recurrent cases can be made much earlier, at about 16 weeks. In that case, for many couples, PGD would be less attractive, since prenatal diagnosis would enable them to make a more informed reproductive decision. In our opinion, both options seem to be morally justified: parents should be allowed to opt for the alternative that suits them best.

Holt–Oram syndrome (HOS)   HOS is a familial heart–hand syndrome characterized by congenital heart malformation in the setting of upper-limb malformation. The penetrance of this syndrome is apparently complete, but the expression is highly variable. In some cases, the spectrum may result in just a minor malformation of the thumb.

Prenatal diagnosis of HOS at the DNA level allows detection of the mutation. HOS has been shown to result from mutations in different genes and from different mutations within the same gene. It would be fine if it was possible to use this genetic heterogeneity to predict genotype/phenotype correlations. Germ-line mutations of the TBX5 gene were identified as the primary cause in up to 70% of patients with HOS[17]. Basson *et al.* studied the clinical features of HOS caused by ten different TBX5 mutations[18]. So-called null alleles caused substantial abnormalities in both limb and heart. In contrast, missense mutations produced distinct phenotypes: significant cardiac malformations but only minor skeletal abnormalities were found in some, whereas others produced extensive upper-limb malformations but less significant cardiac abnormalities. However, Brassington *et al.* concluded that the type of mutation in TBX5 is not predictive of the expressivity of malformations in individuals with HOS[19]. As far as ultrasonographic prenatal diagnosis of HOS is concerned, there is not a large body of literature. However, it seems possible to exclude early in gestation the more severe forms of HOS, whereas small cardiac malformations such as some atrial septal defects, can only be detected in the third trimester[20].

Recent publications suggest that PGD may be a viable alternative[13,21]. PGD seems to be justified, in view of the high penetrance of the relevant mutations and the severity of the symptoms in many cases, even though prenatal ultrasound could give more precise information regarding fetal skeletal and cardiac anatomy in each individual case.

Non-syndromal cleft lip and palate (CL/P)   PGD for genetic susceptibilities to (non-syndromal) CL/P is, for the moment, a purely theoretical option, but this might change in the future. It is to be expected that this case would be highly controversial, both for deontological/ethical and for more practical (technical) reasons. The former can be illustrated by the debate about prenatal diagnosis and possible selective abortion; there is major opposition to selective abortion in these cases, mainly because (non-syndromal) CL/P is often considered as largely cosmetic, and reconstructive surgery usually has good results. In fact, the case of selective abortion because of CL/P often functions as a paradigmatic case of 'misuse of prenatal diagnosis'.

In view of the generally good outcome of treatment of CL/P, it is widely – and rightly – felt that the establishment of optimism and hope around a craniofacial diagnosis is a critical step in starting the process of treatment and care, even during the prenatal period[22]. For the large majority of prospective parents at risk of having a child with CL/P, selective abortion is not an acceptable option. According to a recent survey in Argentina, the majority of parents of children with non-syndromal oral clefts do not consider this to be a serious condition[23]. The authors comment, however, that only one-third of them would have more children if the recurrence risk were as low as 5%. In view of this overall positive picture, a publication from Israel which reports that, in a series of 15 cases of cleft lip detected during routine ultrasound, 14 cases were terminated, caused considerable concern[24,25]. After all, this is at odds with clinical practice and experience in other countries/centers. Commentators doubted, for instance, whether the quality of the counseling was adequate.

While we share these commentators' concerns, we wonder whether a categorical, a priori moral rejection of selective abortion because of CL/P is justified, as it may not fully do justice to the burdens involved for both affected children and their parents. After all, the medical management of the defect often takes many years, and entails a cascade of surgical interventions, especially in the case of cleft lip *and palate*. Furthermore, a cleft palate may cause functional impairments. There may also be significant psychological burdens for affected children. While, according to a recent systematic review, the majority of children and adults with CL/P do not appear to experience major psychosocial problems, problems may arise. For example, difficulties have been reported in relation to behavioral problems, satisfaction with facial appearance, depression and anxiety. A few differences between cleft types have been found in relation to self-concept, satisfaction with facial appearance, depression, attachment, learning problems and interpersonal relationships[26].

Apart from the psychosocial impact of CL/P for affected children themselves, there may be substantial emotional burdens for the parents, especially for parents who grew up with CL/P themselves and for whom this was a traumatic experience (personal communication, Dr Chris Verhaak). In individual cases, they find the possible confrontation with the same handicap in their future child unbearable. For these parents, just taking the recurrence risk is not an option. In view of this, we doubt whether prenatal diagnosis and selective abortion in these cases is, a priori, morally unacceptable. Needless to say, pre- and post-test counseling is crucially important in order to contribute to well-considered decisions.

Should, then, PGD be considered in the case of a higher risk of non-syndromal CL/P? In the context of PGD, additional problems to be addressed are, to a large degree, of a more practical kind. In view of the multifactorial nature of CL/P, the recurrence risk usually is only 3–5%. The predictive value of a possible positive DNA test would be low. To perform IVF/PGD because of a 3–5% recurrence risk of having a child affected with CL/P would be disproportionate. In rare cases, however, the recurrence risk may be substantially higher, maybe up to 50% (see www.ncbi.nlm.nih.gov/entrez/dispomim.cgi?id=119570). Could IVF/PGD, then, be acceptable in these unusual cases? This question may become particularly relevant for the clinic if ongoing research were to clarify further genotype–phenotype correlations, providing more precise information about specific mutations which imply substantially increased risks for cleft lip *and palate*. The outcome of weighing the pros and cons of possible future PGD for CL/P will also be influenced by new insights regarding *primary prevention* of non-syndromal CL/P – or at least risk reduction – by, for instance, periconceptional folic acid supplementation. Clearly, the more effective these strategies prove to be, the less acceptable PGD will be.

If PGD for CL/P were, in rare cases, to be considered a possible option in the future, again, adequate counseling would be of paramount importance. (Prospective) parents should be informed that prenatal ultrasound detection of a cleft lip (at approximately 20 weeks of gestation) will enable them to make better-informed decisions.

Childhood disorders

Difficult questions may also present themselves regarding PGD for childhood disorders caused by less penetrant genes. Relevant cases might concern, for example, cardiovascular disorders, such as long-QT syndrome (LQTS). LQTS mutations regularly have a penetrance of approximately 50%. As we have not yet seen real cases in this field, we briefly tick off a case regarding 'juvenile' diabetes.

Type 1 diabetes The difficulties of PGD for susceptibilities such as type 1 diabetes can be illustrated using a case from Brussels Academic Hospital. A couple having a child severely affected with type 1 diabetes applied for PGD. It was estimated, taking into account possible HLA haplotype combinations, that 25% of their next children would have a 15–20% risk to develop type 1 diabetes, while the remaining 75% would have a risk of approximately 5%.

After extensive deliberations, the ethics committee was undecided about whether or not to perform IVF/PGD in this situation. The case was complicated by both the a priori risk and the significant residual risk. IVF/PGD in order to achieve a risk reduction of 10–15% in one in four embryos seems to be problematic, given the medical, emotional and financial burden of an IVF treatment, the workload of IVF/PGD clinics and the significant residual risks (approximately 5%). But how does one decide if the residual risk is only 1–2% in individual cases?

Adult-onset disorders

PGD – like prenatal diagnosis – for late-onset disorders is especially controversial. The British Medical Association (BMA) has concerns about the routine use of prenatal diagnosis for adult-onset disorders, but accepts that in some circumstances such testing could be appropriate[27]. Unfortunately, the BMA does not clarify whether it has the same concerns about *PGD* for these disorders, thereby suggesting that the criteria may be somewhat less strict in this context. Some commentators consider both prenatal diagnosis and PGD for late-onset disorders to be unjustified[28]. Taking Huntington's disease (HD) as a paradigm case, these critics object that the child will have many decades of good and unimpaired living, and that the parents are not immediately affected in the way that they would be were the disease of early onset. We should, so the critique runs, acknowledge the moral ambiguity of the 'quest for perfect babies' and resist the 'tyranny of the normal'. These objections are, however, not convincing. It is difficult to see why carriers of HD at 50% risk of transmitting the HD mutation to their children would not have the right to prevent this by using modern technology[1,10]. A basic error is, we think, these critics' suggestion that late-onset disorders constitute a homogeneous category of disorders. They ignore the relevance of variables such as the severity of the various disorders, the penetrance of the mutations and the potential availability of preventive and/or therapeutic measures. In view of these variables, PGD for HD may well be the simple case of PGD for late-onset disorders. After all, the penetrance of the genetic defect is complete, and the disorder is lethal. Likewise, PGD (and prenatal testing) for Li–Fraumeni syndrome (LFS) – a dominantly inherited tumor syndrome – seems to be morally justified; tumors sometimes manifest themselves already at a young age, are often difficult to treat and in many cases are even lethal. Furthermore, the penetrance of the causative p53 mutation is very high, if not complete[29]. Far more controversial is (prenatal diagnosis and) PGD of hereditary breast and ovarian cancer, caused by mutations in breast cancer genes called BRCA-1 and -2. A statement of the Dutch Association of Clinical Genetics, to give just one example, concluding that prenatal testing for BRCA-1 or -2 is not a priori ethically unacceptable, caused considerable debate[30].

Hereditary breast and ovarian cancer (HBOC) A preliminary issue regarding PGD concerns the possible health risks of IVF, particularly the hormones given, for female carriers of mutations in BRCA. Recent research suggests that these treatments may carry somewhat higher health risks for these women[31]. Some clinics may, therefore, decide not to perform IVF in these women. Others will conclude, for the moment, that more data are needed, and that women should be able to decide for themselves, after adequate counseling. The latter policy seems to be acceptable from a moral point of view. Clearly, in the case of *male* carriers of BRCA mutations, this issue if irrelevant. What, then, about PGD?

Critics usually have two objections: first, the penetrance of BRCA-1/-2 mutations is incomplete; and second, preventive interventions may effectively reduce morbidity and mortality in (female) carriers[32,33]. We doubt whether these objections are convincing. After all, while the penetrance of BRCA mutations is indeed incomplete, it is still (very) high. Although the relevant publications show considerable variation regarding risk percentages, risks may (according to the guidance used in Dutch clinical genetics centers) be summarized as follows:

(1) Risk of female carriers of a mutation in BRCA-1/-2 to develop breast cancer before the age of 70: 60–80%;

(2) Risk of female carriers of a mutation in BRCA-1 to develop ovarian cancer before the age of 70: 30–60%;

(3) Risk of female carriers of a mutation in BRCA-2 to develop ovarian cancer before the age of 70: 5–20%.

Furthermore, critics of (prenatal diagnosis and) PGD of mutations in BRCA tend to sketch a rather optimistic picture regarding (female) carriers' preventive and therapeutic options. Relevant questions concern the effectiveness of these options, as well as the burden imposed by the respective medical interventions. Unfortunately, the effectiveness of medical surveillance of the breasts is, to date, far from optimal. Maybe magnetic resonance imaging (MRI) will increase the sensitivity of this surveillance and contribute to a reduction of mortality in female carriers[34]. Although the effectiveness of prophylactic mastectomy appears to be high, longer follow-up studies and study of more carriers are necessary to establish definitively the protective value (and determine the long-term complications) of this procedure[35,36]. Furthermore, prophylactic surgery is irreversible, and may have major implications for women's quality of life. The latter are often underestimated[37]. Finally, periodic examination of the ovaries has not been proved effectively to reduce mortality in carriers of BRCA mutations.

In view of this, we would argue that the fear of prospective parents that their future daughter may inherit the mutation is far from unreasonable, and that PGD is justified[38].

CONCLUSIONS AND RECOMMENDATIONS

The practice of both prenatal diagnosis and PGD is dynamic, as the list of defects which can be diagnosed constantly grows longer. The question 'where to draw the line?' is, not surprisingly, among the hot topics in bioethical debates. Focusing on the ethics of PGD for disorders that do not follow simple Mendelian inheritance patterns, we have come to the following conclusions:

(1) Even though PGD for susceptibilities for these disorders raises troubling questions, it cannot be categorically dismissed on ethical grounds. To argue that PGD should only be performed if the penetrance of the specific mutation is almost complete is too restrictive and is at odds with current clinical practice, namely PGD for medical sex selection. After all, the risk for male embryos/future boys is 'just' 50%.

(2) Morally relevant variables to be taken into account include, apart from the personal situation/history of the individual applicants: the severity of the disorder, the penetrance of the mutation, the age of onset of the disorder, the availability of measures for primary prevention and the possible residual risks for the future child.

(3) Adequate counseling, aiming at informed choice, is a prerequisite. Clients should understand that, especially for congenital malformations, regular prenatal diagnosis (especially ultrasound) may be far more informative than PGD. However, in some cases this information might become available only late in pregnancy, which might hamper a decision in favor of pregnancy termination.

A further debate is, no doubt, necessary. Many difficult cases will come to the fore, including cases regarding kinds of disorders that have, so far, not been tested for. While, according to the Nuffield Council on Bioethics, prenatal and preimplantation testing for the common mental disorders is unlikely to have sufficient predictive value to be indicated or to be demanded by prospective parents, there may well be exceptions to this rule, especially when higher-penetrance susceptibilities might be found in the future[39]: *festina lente*.

REFERENCES

1. De Wert G. Ethical aspects of prenatal testing and preimplantation genetic testing for late-onset neurogenetic disease: the case of Huntington's disease. In Evers-Kiebooms G, Zoeteweij M, Harper PS, eds. Prenatal Testing for Late-onset Neurogenetic Diseases. Oxford: BIOS, 2002: 129–58.
2. Steinbock B. Preimplantation genetic diagnosis and embryo selection. In: Burley C, Harris J, eds. A Companion to Genethics. Malden, USA: Blackwell, 2002: 147–57.
3. De Wert G. Met het oog op de toekomst. Voortplantingsgeneeskunde, erfelijkheidsonderzoek en ethiek. Amsterdam: Thela Thesis, 1999.
4. Robertson JA. Ethical and legal issues in preimplantation genetic screening. Fertil Steril 1992; 57: 1–11.
5. Shenfield F, Pennings G, Devroey P, et al. The ESHRE Ethics Task Force. Preimplantaton genetic diagnosis. Hum Reprod 2003; 18: 649–51.
6. Strong, C. Ethics in reproductive and Perinatal Medicine. A New Framework. New Haven: Yale University Press, 1997.

7.   Andrews LB, Fullarton JE, Holtzman NA, Motulsky AG, eds. Assessing Genetic Risks. Implications for Health and Social Policy. Washington, DC: National Academy Press, 1994.

8.   Royal Commission on New Reproductive Technologies. Proceed with Care. Ottawa: Minister of Government Services Canada, 1993.

9.   Steinbock B. Prenatal genetic testing for Alzheimer's disease. In Post SG, Whitehouse PJ, eds. Genetic Testing for Alzheimer Disease. Ethical and Clinical Issues. Baltimore, MD: John Hopkins University Press, 1998: 140–51.

10.   De Wert G. Prenatale diagnostiek en selectieve abortus. Enkele ethische overwegingen. In Ten Have H, et al., eds. Ethiek en recht in de gezondheidszorg, Deel XVI. Lochem: De Tijdstroom, 1990: 121–53.

11.   American Medical Association. Council on Ethical and Judicial Affairs. Ethical issues related to prenatal genetic testing. Arch Fam Med 1994; 3: 633–42.

12.   Pennings G. Personal desires of patients and social obligations of geneticists: applying preimplantation genetic diagnosis for non-medical sex selection. Prenat Diagn 2002; 22: 1123–9.

13.   He J, McDermott DA, Song Y, et al. Preimplantation genetic diagnosis of human congenital heart malformation and Holt–Oram syndrome. Am J Med Genet 2004; 126A: 93–8.

14.   Verlinsky Y, Rechitsky S, Verlinsky O, et al. Preimplantation diagnosis for sonic hedgehog mutation causing familial holoprosencephaly. N Engl J Med 2003; 348: 1449–54.

15.   Lai T-H, Chang C-H, Yu C-H, et al. Prenatal diagnosis of alobar holoprosencephaly by two-dimensional and three-dimensional ultrasound. Prenat Diagn 2000; 20: 400–3.

16.   Chen C-P, Shih J-C, Hsu C-Y, et al. Prenatal three-dimensional/four-dimensional sonographic demonstration of facial dysmorphisms associated with holoprosencephaly. J Clin Ultrasound 2005; 33: 312–18.

17.   Heinritz W, Shou L, Moschik A, Froster UG. The human TBX5 gene mutation database. Hum Mutat 2005; 26: 397.

18.   Basson CT, Huang T, Lin RC, et al. Different TBX5 interactions in heart and limb defined by Holt–Oram syndrome mutations. Proc Natl Acad Sci USA 1999; 96: 2919–24.

19.   Brassington AM, Sung SS, Toydemir RM, et al. Expressivity of Holt–Oram syndrome is not predicted by TBX5 genotype. Am J Hum Genet 2003; 73: 74–85.

20.   Brons JT, Van Geijn HP, Wladimiroff J, et al. Prenatal ultrasound diagnosis of the Holt–Oram syndrome. Prenat Diagn 1988; 8: 175–81.

21.   McDermott AD, He J, Song YS, et al. Update: PGD and Holt–Oram sydrome. Am J Med Genet 2005; 136A: 223.

22.   Strauss RP. Beyond easy answers: prenatal diagnosis and counselling during pregnancy. Cleft-Palate Craniofac J 2002; 39: 164–86.

23.   Wyszynski DF, Perandones C, Bennun RD. Attitudes toward prenatal diagnosis, termination of pregnancy, and reproduction by parents of children with non-syndromic oral clefts in Argentina. Prenat Diagn 2003; 23: 722–7.

24.   Bronshtein M, Blumenfeld I, Blumenfeld Z. Early prenatal diagnosis of cleft lip and its potential impact on the number of babies with cleft lip. Br J Oral Maxillofac Surg 1996; 34: 486–7.

25. Strauss RP. Ethical issues in the care of children with craniofacial conditions. In: Wyszynski DF, ed. Cleft Lip and Palate. From Origin to Treatment. New York: Oxford University Press, 2002: 481–7.

26. Hunt O, Burden D, Hepper P, Johnston C. The psychosocial effects of cleft lip and palate: a systematic review. Eur J Orthodont 2005; 27: 274–85.

27. British Medical Association Ethics Department. Medical Ethics Today. The BMA's Handbook of Ethics and Law. London: BMA, 2003.

28. Post S. Selective abortion and gene therapy: reflections on human limits. Hum Gene Ther 1991; 2: 229–33.

29. Verlinsky Y, Rechitsky S, Verlinsky O, et al. Preimplantation diagnosis for p53 tumor suppressor gene mutations. Reprod Biomed Online 2001; 2: 102–5.

30. Cobben JM, Broecker-Vriends AHJT, Leschot NJ. Prenatale diagnostiek naar de erfelijke aanleg voor mamma-/ovariumcarcinoom – een standpuntbepaling. Ned Tijdschr Geneeskd 2002; 146: 1461–5.

31. Friedman LC, Kramer RM. Reproductive issues for women with BRCA mutations. J Natl Cancer Inst Monogr 2005; 34: 83–6.

32. Lancaster JM, Wiseman RW, Berchuck A. An inevitable dilemma. Obstet Gynecol 1996; 87: 306–9.

33. Wagner TMU, Ahner R. Prenatal testing for late-onset diseases such as mutations in the breast cancer gene 1 (BRCA 1). Hum Reprod 1998; 13: 1125–8.

34. Kriege M, Brekelmans CT, Boetes C, et al. Magnetic resonance imaging screening study group. Efficacy of MRI and mammography for breast-cancer screening in women with a familial or genetic predisposition. N Engl J Med 2004; 351: 427–37.

35. Meijers-Heijboer H, Van Geel B, Van Putten W, et al. Breast cancer after prophylactic bilateral mastectomy in women with a BRCA1 or BRCA2 mutation. N Engl J Med 2001; 345: 159–64.

36. Lostumbo L, Carbine N, Wallace J, Ezzo J. Prophylactic mastectomy for the prevention of breast cancer. Cochrane Database Syst Rev 2004; (4): CD002748.

37. Van Oostrom I, Meijers-Heijboer H, Lodder LN, et al. Long-term psychological impact of carrying a BRCA1/2 mutation and prophylactic surgery: a 5-year follow-up study. J Clin Oncol 2003; 21: 3867–74.

38. De Wert G. Ethics of predictive DNA-testing for hereditary breast and ovarian cancer. Patient Educ Counsel 1998; 35: 43–52.

39. Nuffield Council on Bioethics. Mental Disorders and Genetics: the Ethical Context. London: Nuffield Council on Bioethics, 1998.

Chapter 8

Religious perspectives on ethical issues in assisted reproductive technologies

Gamal I Serour

RELIGIOUS PERSPECTIVES ON ETHICAL ISSUES IN ART

'Science without conscience ruins the soul'[1]. It is therefore not surprising that science and religion have been inter-related since the beginning of human history, although the past four decades have witnessed the secularization of bioethics. This has led to a subsequent decline of religious influence in the field of ethics, which has become dominated by philosophical, social and legal concepts[2]. However, in some parts of the world such as the Middle East, from where the three major religions, namely Judaism, Christianity and Islam, emerged, religion is still meaningful and influences many behaviors, practices and policies. This also applies to conservative followers of these religions in different parts of the world. All three major religions have encouraged procreation within the frame of marriage.

In Judaism, marriage is both a religious and a legal act between a man and his chosen mate, and is considered to be one of the most useful means of preventing sexual sins, and the proper way to fulfill God's commandment: 'Be fruitful, and multiply'[3]. The most striking development in the evolution of Christianity from its Jewish origin has been the transition from a national religion (of the Jewish nation) to a universal religion. Issues of sexuality, marriage and parenthood are also central to Christian values. Christians were heirs to the Greeks as well as to the Jews. From them, Christians learned that moral theory must relate to facts, to reality as known.

Influenced by Greek science, rabbis in Alexandria included in the Greek (Septuagint) version of Exodus the principle that protection due to the embryo/fetus advances step by step with its morphological development and growth. This was then integrated into Christian philosophy, theology, morality and canon law, and hence also into the common law. This 'gradualism' was the standard assumption and teaching in the Roman Catholic Church virtually until 1869, when Pope Pius IX ended it in favor of absolute protection from the moment of conception.

Similarly, the Holy Qur'an encouraged marriage, family formation and reproduction, saying: 'We did send apostles, before thee, and appointed for them wives and children'[4].

Other traditions also place special emphasis on reproduction. In Chinese culture, the universe is an organism which is capable of continuous reproduction, transformation and creation. It is said that 'all things are created by intercourse between male and female': if there had been no intercourse between heaven and earth, there would not have been all things in the world[5]. Traditional Chinese culture emphasizes the importance of having many children and continuation of the male family line[6]. Confucians believe that the function of sex is reproduction, and childlessness means an incomplete or less than perfect family. Taoists believe that sex is indispensable for human life and health.

Amongst the Hindu, kinship and family ties depend on progeny. A woman is considered 'complete' or 'real' only when she becomes a mother. Fertility defines womanhood, and womanhood is defined by a woman's capacity to 'mother'. Thus, society puts pressure on her to become a mother even though the male partner may be infertile.

With the advent of assisted reproductive technologies (ART) with the birth of Louise Brown in the UK on 25th July 1978, it became possible to separate the bonding of reproduction from the sexual act[7]. ART, whether *in vivo* or *in vitro*, enabled women to conceive without having intercourse. ART also allowed the involvement of a third party in the process of reproduction whether by providing an egg, a sperm, an embryo or a uterus, and also opened the way for several other practices including gender selection, preimplantation genetic diagnosis (PGD), genetic manipulation, cryopreservation of gametes, embryos and gonads, cloning, etc. This challenged age-old ideas and provoked ethical debate which has continued since the earliest days[8].

Principles such as the 'sanctity of life' may be absolute, or given a high but presumptive value – thus opening the door for moral reasoning to establish the limits of liberty[9]. With globalization, doctors and patients alike are moving around to different parts of the world, and it may not be uncommon that physicians provide medical services to patients with ethical values different from their own. It becomes therefore mandatory to be aware of various religious perspectives on various practices in ART.

JEWISH PERSPECTIVES ON ETHICAL ISSUES IN ART

A strict association between faith and practical rules characterizes the Jewish religion. Jewish law has two sources: written law (the Torah) and verbal law. The Torah is viewed as a single unit, a divine text that includes moral values as well as practical laws (first five books of scriptures), whilst verbal laws interpret, expand and elucidate the written Torah and include the Mishnah (third century), followed three centuries later by the Talmud (and its code Halakha), and finally

Post-Talmudic Codes (16th century) or Responsa, the term confined to written replies given by rabbinical scholars to questions on all aspects of Jewish law, including questions on ART. Some individual rabbis have taken a strict position, and suggested that legal and biological ties be severed with removal of the egg from the body, but both chief Rabbis of Israel (of Ashkenazi or European origin and Sephardic/Oriental origin) support ART. At a worldwide level, there are several different trends in Judaism: the orthodox group which constitute about 10% of religious Jews, whilst reform (introduced by German Jews in the 1830s) and conservative (which began in 1887 as a counter-reform) account for, respectively, 85% and 5% of religious Jews. The reform movement leadership agreed in 1952 that all efforts should be made to help the infertile, whilst conservative Judaism, which mostly expanded during and after the horrors of World War II, showed from its earliest days a willingness to respond to contemporary issues. Thus, for most groups, embryo research is acceptable, as until 40 days after conception the fertilized egg is considered mere fluid[10], with no moral status for the embryo.

In general, there is near unanimity of opinion that the use of semen from the husband is permissible if no other method is possible for the wife to become pregnant. Masturbation should be avoided if at all possible, and coitus interruptus or the use of a perforated condom seems to be the preferred method for provision of sperm

Sperm donation is, however, generally prohibited because of fear of incest, prohibition of masturbation, disturbance of genealogy and possible problems of inheritance. All orthodox Jewish legal experts agree that sperm donation using the semen of a Jewish donor is forbidden, but some rabbinical authorities (reform and conservative) permit sperm donation when the donor is a non-Jew, and absolve the woman from adultery. Egg donation is acceptable, as only the offspring of a Jewish mother may be regarded as a Jew. Interestingly, in the state of Israel, where much law stems from religious Jewish orthodoxy but where probably 50% of citizens are not religious or are of a different faith, donation is also permitted for single women. Oocytes obtained from an unmarried woman and cryopreserved can be donated after her death to another woman if her consent was obtained before her death. Cryopreservation of embryos is permitted with the consent of the parents for a period of 5 years, which is renewable if requested by the couple, but their donation is forbidden. In case of death of the husband (or of divorce), the embryos may be transferred to the wife within 1 year after death of her husband, if supported by the recommendation of a social worker (or written permission in the case of divorce).

Jewish religion does not forbid the practice of surrogacy, whether complete or partial, as indeed the practice is described in the Bible in the case of Sarah and Abram, with Hagar who bore Abram a son, Ishmael, and Rachel, who used her slave-girl Bilha to bear a child for Jacob[11,12]. Based on the biblical precedents, various practices of surrogacy available today are therefore acceptable.

In the state of Israel, the 'Approving Committee' must authorize every single case of surrogacy. This multidisciplinary committee nominated by the Health

Minister includes an obstetrician and gynecologist, physician, clinical psychologist, social worker, lawyer and clergyman according to the religion of the parties involved, and takes a majority decision.

Finally, consider the dilemmas of fetal reduction, sex selection and cloning.

Halachic authorities would allow fetal reduction, if it is absolutely certain that all fetuses would be lost otherwise and if prevention fails, in cases of high-order multiple pregnancy.

In traditional Jewish law, sons are important for religious reasons. After the death of a parent, the son says the Kaddish (prayer) for the dead[10]. Recently, the state of Israel issued a legislation giving state support for an *in vitro* fertilization (IVF) cycle with sex selection for families who have four or more children of the same sex and wish for a child of the other sex.

A minority of Jewish scholars do not believe that potential violations of human dignity are reason enough to prohibit human cloning[13], and regard cloning of a family member as more acceptable than donor insemination or egg donation, but other Jewish thinkers oppose reproductive cloning, because it might harm the family by changing the roles and relationships between members. Indeed, Israel was one of the first countries to adopt in 1998 a law that prohibits reproductive cloning. This moratorium was extended for an additional 5 years by the Knesset in 2004[14].

CHRISTIAN PERSPECTIVES ON ETHICAL ISSUES IN ART

Christianity is centered on Jesus, the Son of God, and his supreme revelation. Christian beliefs are based on his teachings, as reported in the four officially accepted Gospels, and on the Jewish Scriptures, which Christians call the Old Testament. When some principles are given absolute value in an authoritarian community, prohibitions follow. This is illustrated in the Catholic tradition, where the 'sanctity of life' is considered absolute 'from the moment of fertilization', forbidding IVF, embryo research and PGD. It is difficult to find common elements, other than origin and the acceptance of common sacred writings and symbols among all Christian churches. Indeed, Christianity does not speak with one voice on ART. The Catholic view from Rome, putting an absolute value on the unbreakable nexus between coitus and conception, forbids all members any ART practice which bypasses the sexual union of man and woman[15]. Although marriage confers upon the spouses the right to perform the natural acts of conjugal love which aim at procreation, the child is not an object, but the most gratuitous gift of marriage[16].

In the Protestant churches, moral reasoning is the perennial task, establishing the acceptable limits in the application of new developments in science and technology, including ART[9]. It is thought that infertile people have a proper claim on medical technology, and must be informed and counseled as they are vulnerable and therefore prone to exploitation. Thus, The Kirk (the Church of Scotland) allows embryo research, whilst being opposed to any extension of the 14-day limit. Like the Church of England, it does not impose these judgments on members as matters of strict obedience or prohibition, but issues them as guidelines for making their own judgments in conscience. The Anglican Church is liberal on the use of ART, and allows semen collection by means of masturbation. However, it forbids the use of donor gametes. In May 1996, the General Assembly of the Church of Scotland (The Kirk) expressed its agreement that ART may be appropriate for married couples and even for unmarried couples living in a stable and long-lasting relationship. It is opposed to the donation of sperm and of ova, surrogacy and sex selection, except to prevent the transmission of inherited disease[17].

Many other Protestant churches would allow ART with spouse gametes and no embryo wastage. The Eastern Orthodox Church supports medical and surgical treatment of infertility including ART, but not gamete donation or surrogacy, like the Church of Alexandria[18].

With regard to the specific problem of multiple pregnancy, in spite of the recognized maternal and fetal risks, Pope John Paul II in an encyclical letter to all Catholics warned in 1995 of the rise of a 'culture of death' in modern society, using his strongest language to condemn abortion, which he described as a crime which no human law can claim to legitimize. Thus, according to Catholic faith, multifetal pregnancy reduction cannot be legitimized, even though it does not intend to induce abortion.

It also prohibits any destruction of embryos to favor the birth of one sex or the other, whether for medical or social reason it is forbidden, by whatever method, from microsort sperm separation technique to PGD.

But in societies where Christianity has been historically the majority denomination, sex-selection technologies for disease preventions are generally allowed, and their use for social indications has led to a great deal of ethical debate[19]. Interest in sex selection for social indications is not new in Europe: Millot, the obstetrician of Queen Marie Antoinette of France (1820), wrote, 'it is the last movement of the woman that determines the sex of the child: it is the side on which she lies at ejaculation time that drives to sex of the child: always a boy when she is on the right side and always a girl on the left side'[20]. Recent studies have shown that Europeans would choose to have a baby regardless of whether sex selection was possible or not[21]. In the UK, over half of surveyed couples selecting their children's sex chose girls[22]. However, a public consultation on social sex selection conducted by the Human Fertilisation and Embryology Authority revealed that 69% of respondents rejected the principle, a decline from 80% in 1993[23]. In Canada, a national survey of preferences regarding the sex of children showed that a large majority do not prefer children of one sex or the other[24], but would like at least one child of each sex. Sons are preferred as first-born children among parents with a sex preference, but the majority of zero-parity women have no sex preference for their first-born child[25]. Finally, gender selection for non-medical reasons has been practiced in the United States for decades, but is uncommon in Australia.

In the document: 'Donum vitae', Roman Catholics were told that cloning was considered contrary to moral law, since it is in opposition to the dignity both of human procreation and of the conjugal union. Methods that fail to respect the dignity and value of the person must always be avoided. Attempts at human cloning with a view to obtaining tissues/organs for transplants, in so far as they involve the manipulation and destruction of human embryos, are not morally acceptable even when their proposed goal is good in itself[26].

These prohibitive instructions are not only restricted to the Catholic Church. Indeed, some Evangelical churches are equally authoritative in their prohibitions.

ISLAMIC PERSPECTIVES ON ETHICAL ISSUES IN ART

The teaching of Islam covers all fields of human activity: spiritual and material, individual and social, educational and cultural, economic and political, national and international. The instruction which regulates everyday activities of life to be adhered to by good Muslims is called Sharia. There are two sources of Sharia in Islam: primary and secondary. The primary sources of Sharia in chronological order are: the Holy Qur'an, the very word of God; the Sunna and Hadith, which include the authentic traditions and sayings of the Prophet Muhammad as collected by specialists in Hadith; Igmaah, which is the unanimous opinion of Islamic scholars or Aimma; and analogy (Kias), which is the intelligent reasoning used to rule on events not mentioned by the Qur'an and Sunna, by matching against similar or equivalent events already ruled on. The secondary sources of Sharia are Istihsan, which is the choice of one of several lawful options; views of the Prophet's companions; current local customs if lawful; public welfare; and rulings of previous divine religions if they do not contradict the primary sources of Sharia. A good Muslim resorts to secondary sources of Sharia in matters not dealt with by the primary sources. Even if the action is forbidden, it may be undertaken if the alternative would cause harm. The Sharia is not rigid. It is flexible enough to adapt to emerging situations according to different items and places. It can accommodate various honest opinions as long as they do not conflict with the spirit of its primary sources and are directed toward the benefit of humanity[27,28]. Islam is a religion of Yusr (ease), not Usr (hardship), as indicated in the Holy Qur'an[29]. The broad principles of Islamic jurisprudence are permissibility unless prohibited by a text (Ibaha), no harm and no harassment; necessity permits the prohibited and the choice of the lesser harm. ART was not mentioned in the primary sources of Sharia. However, these same sources have affirmed the importance of marriage, family formation and procreation. Also, in Islam, adoption is not acceptable as a solution to the problem of infertility. Islam gives legal precedence to purity of lineage and known parenthood of all children. The Qur'an explicitly prohibits legal adoption but encourages kind upbringing of orphans[30]. In Islam, treating infertility with permitted techniques is allowed and encouraged. It is essential if it involves preservation of procreation and treatment of infertility in married couples[27]. This is applicable to ART, which is one line of treatment of infertility. The prevention and treatment of infertility are of particular significance in the Muslim world, as the social status of Muslim women, their dignity and their self-esteem are closely related to their procreation potential, both for the family and for society as a whole; childbirth and -rearing are regarded as family commitments and not just biological and social functions. As ART was not mentioned in the primary sources of Sharia, patients and Muslim doctors alike initially thought that seeking ART was a challenge to God's will by trying to render barren women fertile, and by handling human gametes and embryos. ART was only widely accepted after prestigious scientific and religious bodies and organizations issued guidelines which were adopted by Medical Councils or concerned authorities in different Muslim countries and which controlled the practices in ART centers.

These guidelines, which played a role in a change of attitude of both society and individuals in the Muslim world, included a Fatwa from Al-Azhar, Cairo (1980)[31], and Fatwa from the Islamic Fikh Council, Mecca (1984)[32], the Organization of Islamic Medicine in Kuwait (1991), Qatar University (1993), the Islamic Education, science and culture organization in Rabaat (2002), the United Arab Emirates (2002) and the International Islamic Center for Population Studies and Research at Al-Azhar University[33-37]. These bodies stressed the fact that Islam encouraged marriage, family formation and procreation in its primary sources. Treatment of infertility, including ART when indicated, is encouraged to preserve humankind within the frame of marriage, in otherwise incurable infertility. The attitude of patients changed from rejection, doubt and feelings of shame, guilt and secrecy when requesting ART in the 1980s to openly seeking ART in the 1990s. The introduction of effective intracytoplasmic sperm injection (ICSI) treatment for male infertility played a role in the change of attitude of many couples to ART[28]. In family affairs, particularly reproduction, decisions are usually taken by the couple, but not uncommonly, the husband's decision is prevalent. Husbands became very enthusiastic about ART. They took the initiative and encouraged their wives to undergo ART treatment for male, female or unexplained infertility. Today, the basic guidelines for ART in the Muslim world are: if ART is indicated in a married couple as a necessary line of treatment it is permitted during validity of the marriage contract with no mixing of genes. If the marriage contract has come to an end because of divorce or death of the husband, artificial reproduction cannot be performed in the female partner, even using sperm cells from her former husband. The Shi'aa guidelines have 'opened' the way to third-party donation, via a Fatwa from Ayatollah Ali Hussein Khomeini in 1999. This Fatwa allowed third-party participation including egg donation, sperm donation and surrogacy, and is gaining acceptance in parts of the Shi'ite world. Recently, there has been some concern about sperm donation among Shi'aa. All these practices of third-party participation in reproduction are based on the importance of maintaining the family structure and integrity among the Shi'aa family. They are allowed within various temporary marriage contract arrangements with the concerned donors.

Surrogacy

Surrogacy is not permitted for most Sunni. The Fatwa of the Fikh Council in 1984 allowed surrogacy by replacing the embryos inside the uterus of the second wife of the same husband who provided the sperm. In 1985, the Council withdrew its approval of surrogacy, but the debate has recently been re-opened among Sunni scholars. While some religious authorities think that it can be permitted, others believe that it should not be approved.

Cryopreservation

The excess number of fertilized eggs can be preserved by cryoperservation. The frozen embryos are the property of the couple alone, and may be transferred to the same wife in a successive cycle but only during the validity of the marriage contract[34-36]. Whether a couple's preserved embryos could be implanted in a wife after her husband's death was discussed in an international workshop organized by The International Islamic Center for Population Studies and Research, Al-Azhar University, in 2000. The strict view was that marriage ends at death, and procuring pregnancy in an unmarried woman is forbidden by religious laws, for instance regarding children's rights to be reared by two parents, and regarding inheritance. After due time, the widow might remarry, but could not then bear a child that was not her new husband's. An opposing view, advanced as reflecting both Islamic compassion and women's interests as widows, was that a woman left alone through early widowhood would be well and tolerably served by bearing her deceased husband's child, through her enjoying companionship, discharge of religious duties of child-rearing and later support. The Grand Mufti of Egypt (personal communication) stated that permission had once been given for embryo implantation in a wife following her husband's death, based on the circumstances of the particular case. However, this should not be taken as a generalization, and each case should be considered on its own merits[36-38].

Multifetal pregnancy reduction

Multifetal pregnancy, particularly high-order multiple pregnancy (HOMP), should be prevented in the first place. Should HOMP occur in spite of all preventive measures, then multifetal pregnancy reduction may be performed, and applying the jurisprudence principle of necessity permits the prohibited and the choice of the lesser harm. Multifetal pregnancy reduction is only allowed if the prospect of carrying the pregnancy to viability is small. Also, it is allowed if the life or the health of the mother is in jeopardy. It is performed with the intention not to induce abortion but to preserve the life of the remaining fetuses and to minimize complications to the mother[38,39].

Embryo research

According to tradition, the development of the embryo/fetus advances step by step with its morphological development and growth, from a clot, to a lump of flesh, then boned flesh and finally a fully grown infant[40,41]. Until 40 days, the embryo in the mother's womb is a 'nutfa', then an 'alaqa' for an equal period, then a 'mudgha'. Organ differentiation occurs within 42 days after fertilization. Ensoulment of the fetus occurs after 120 days from fertilization[42]. The old threshold of 40 days and upwards from conception has been brought back to 14 days, because the new embryology has established this embryonic period of cellular activity before which individuation cannot begin[33]. Embryo research for the advancement of scientific knowledge and benefit of humanity is therefore allowed before 14 days after fertilization on embryos donated for research with the free, informed consent of the couple. However, these embryos should not be replaced in the uterus of the owner of the eggs or in the uterus of any other woman[31,33,36]. Reflecting the unstructured ethical governance of research in several Muslim countries, each country should form a national research ethics committee to which any proposed research involving the use of gametes or embryos outside the body would be submitted for prior review and approval[38].

Sex selection

Opinion about the use of sperm-sorting techniques or PGD for non-medical reasons such as sex selection or balancing sex ratio in the family is guarded. These techniques are a better alternative to prenatal diagnosis that results in abortion. Muslims adhere to the view that human life requiring protection commences 2–3 weeks from conception and uterine implantation[33]. Accordingly, decisions not to attempt replacement of embryos produced *in vitro* on the grounds that they show serious chromosomal or genetic anomalies, such as aneuploidy, cystic fibrosis, muscular dystrophy or hemophilia, are accepted. PGD is encouraged, where feasible, as an option to avoid clinical pregnancy terminations for couples at exceptionally high risk[38]. More contentious is the non-medical purpose of sex selection. More than 1400 years ago, Arabs before Islam used to practice infanticide for gender selection. The Holy Qur'an described this act and condemned it, stating[43,44]: 'On God's Judgment Day the entombed alive female infant is asked, for what guilt was she made to suffer infanticide?' Sex-selection technologies have been condemned on the basis that their application is to discriminate against female embryos and fetuses, so perpetuating prejudice against the girl child and social devaluation of women[45]. Such discrimination and devaluation are condemned in the Muslim world. However, universal prohibition would itself risk prejudice to women in many present societies, especially while births of sons remain central to women's well-being. Sex-ratio balancing in the family is considered acceptable, for instance where a wife has borne three or four daughters or sons and it is in her and her family's best interests that another pregnancy should be her last. Employing sex-selection techniques to ensure the birth of a son or a daughter might then be approved, to satisfy a sense of religious or family obligation and to save the woman from increasingly risky pregnancies[46-48]. The application of PGD or sperm-sorting techniques for sex selection should be discouraged in principle, but resolved on its particular merits with guidelines to avoid discrimination against either sex, particularly the female child[46]. It should not be used for selection of the sex of the first child or for selection of one sex only in the family. Also, it is only applied to families who have children of one sex and have an intense desire to have one more child of the other sex. The service is provided only after proper counseling with the reproductive-medicine physician, geneticist, social scientist and psychologist.

Pregnancy in the postmenopause

In the past, before cryopreservation was considered, the possibility of postmenopausal pregnancy, dependent on ovum donation, was disapproved in principle as it involves the mixing of genes. Furthermore, pregnancy after the menopause is associated with increased risks for both mother and child. Accordingly, it was unacceptable in the Muslim world[35]. However, with the development of cryopreservation it is now possible to have a pregnancy in the postmenopause using one's own cryopreserved embryos or even oocytes, and, possibly in the future, autografted cryopreserved ovaries. Taking into consideration the special care necessary for the safe induction and completion of pregnancy in a woman who is of advanced, or beyond normal, child-bearing years, the easier case where premature menopause affects a woman who would otherwise be of suitable child-bearing age, and the children's needs for parents likely to survive at least until their mid-adolescence, research efforts should be concentrated on the prevention of premature menopause. Postmenopausal pregnancy in advanced age may be permissible in exceptional cases, justified by the maintenance of integrity of a child's genetic parentage, the pressing nature of the circumstances, the relative safety to mother and child, and the parental capacity to discharge child-rearing responsibilities[38].

Cloning

Reproductive cloning for the creation and birth of a new person who would be the genetic twin of one born previously is condemned. Research into non-reproductive cloning, particularly for stem-cell creation intended for human benefit, is encouraged, whilst recognizing that the use of deliberately created embryos is likely to be involved. Study and research are expected to have a beneficial impact on reproduction, in that the understanding of the origins of genetic defects in embryonic and fetal development would facilitate the prevention and correction of defects, and, when prevention or correction were impossible, the selection of healthy gametes, or embryos. Some theologians are sympathetic to the consideration of reproductive cloning of cells of a childless sterile man with his wife's consent, in order to permit discharge of religious duties, relieve family distress and decrease the risk of marriage breakdown through the wife's right of divorce. On balance, it is considered rather premature to recommend departing from the prevailing condemnation of reproductive cloning[38].

Allied with stem cell research is the prospect of gene therapy. Progress in somatic-cell gene therapy, which alters the genes only of a treated patient, has suffered recent setbacks, and germline gene therapy, which would affect all future generations of a patient's offspring, remains little short of universally condemned and prohibited[49]. Genetic alteration of embryos before their cells have reached differentiation, that is, while they are still totipotent, would need to constitute germline manipulation. Little would be added to reiterate prevailing condemnation. Gene therapy is a developing area that may be used with ART in the future. It is critical that its use be clearly beneficial, focused on alleviating human suffering. The focus on therapeutic applications would exclude purely cosmetic uses and goals of enhancement of non-pathological conditions. Alleviation of genetic diseases and pathological conditions alone would exclude such applications as to make people who would be within the normal range of physique, capacity and aptitude taller, stronger, more likely to achieve athletic success or to be more intelligent or artistically sensitive or gifted. Gene therapy might be legitimate, not to promote advantage or privilege, but to redress genetically or otherwise physiologically inherited disadvantage[27,31,34].

CONFUCIAN–TAOIST AND BUDDHIST PERSPECTIVES ON ETHICAL ISSUES IN ART

Confucianism is mainly a philosophy and ethical code which teaches humans how to be a moral being, as humans are born biologically, but not morally. In Oriental cultures, reproduction is one of the main concerns, linked with the significant value of the family. Filial piety requires people to extend the life of their ancestors and continue the family line from generation to generation. Confucians and Buddhists traditionally considered infertility as a retribution for past immorality of the man, the woman or even their ancestors[50]. Chinese attitudes to infertility and ART are influenced by three values, in ranking order: reproduction, life-preserving or health-promoting and pleasure. In general, any intervention in natural reproduction is undesirable because it disturbs the *dao* of nature, but it is more acceptable than being childless. There are concerns about the environment in which the sperm or the embryo are preserved, and its content of vital energy (*jing* or *yuan qi*), although it cannot be measured. ICSI is not favored because it is thought that in the husband's immature or possibly damaged sperm *yang* or *jing* or *yuan qi* may be deficient, and lead to the birth of an unhealthy child. Although artificial insemination by donor is accepted by traditional Chinese, Chinese men are reluctant to donate sperm because they think that sperm contains *jing* or *yuan qi*, which are indispensable for their health and life. Surrogate motherhood is controversial. Some scholars have suggested a comprehensive ban. Others have opposed this prohibition[51].

Sex selection

In China, there are historical records of the practice of female infanticide[52]. Sons are important for religious reasons, and the traditional family genealogy tree written in ancestral halls records only the names of males, not counting daughters. The traditional cultural norm in old China was to divorce unilaterally women who could not bear a son[53]. The issue of gender preference was complicated by the introduction of the one-child policy: couples in urban areas are usually allowed to have only one child. In rural areas, couples whose first child is a girl may have a second child, but only after a specific time period[54]. Chinese women may want to abort a female fetus so that they may try again for a male child. This practice is leading to a serious imbalance in the sex ratio in China[55]: in some provinces the sex ratio is more than 120 boys for every 100 girls. For all births, there are 113 males for every 100 females.

Sex selection is a symptom of the pervasive social injustice against women, but suppressing the symptom alone leaves substantive injustices unresolved, and may aggravate them by exposing women and girls to the risk of death[56]. Balancing the sex ratio in the family can be accommodated by sex-selection only where a family already has a child, or two or more children of the same sex. Prohibiting sex-selection where discrimination against women and girl children is pervasive is itself insufficient. Rather than resort to criminal law, society at large should tackle the more relevant challenge 'to improve women's social, economic, political and cultural status' in order to eliminate discrimination against women[57].

HINDU PERSPECTIVES ON ETHICAL ISSUES IN ART

There is a huge stigma attached to being infertile in Indian society, especially for the woman[58]. Women go through all kinds of treatments to have a child, because it brings them power in real terms. As ART gives hope to the infertile, even though only a few can afford it, it is perceived as a great scientific achievement among the Hindu. There are no laws regarding the use or standards of ART, donor eggs and sperm, or surrogacy in India.

Patients and physicians alike believe that regulation should be flexible. The recently proposed Indian Council of Medical Research (ICMR) guidelines have generated some interest among practitioners who express both support for efforts to improve safety and concern about the limitations that such restrictions might introduce[59].

With regard to the use of artificial insemination using donor sperm (AID), some report a very marginal acceptance by couples[60], others a tremendous demand for AID[61], or very few couples agreeing to undergo AID[62].

Sex selection

In India, having more than one daughter is a curse, whereas any number of sons is welcomed. Sons are important economically and provide support for aging parents. Until recently, daughters did not have a right to inherit any part of the ancestral or other property of the parents. Further, the traditional practice of dowries continues, in spite of legal prohibition. Thus, a girl child becomes a financial burden on the parents. There are still a number of dowry deaths where the young bride either kills herself or is killed by her in-laws due to disputes about the settlement after marriage. In a few areas, female infanticide is still common practice. All this fuels the desire of many couples to use modern technology to ensure the birth of only a male child, particularly with national policy emphasis on small families[63]. In India, gender selection is blatantly misused to discriminate against female babies. The proportion of females to males dropped from 935 : 1000 in 1981 to 927 : 1000 in 1991. In certain communities in the northern states of Bihar and Rajasthan, the ratio plummeted to 600 : 1000, one of the lowest in the world[64]. The 2001 census of India demonstrated that in the age group of 0–6 years, the sex ratio was 927 females to 1000 males. It was 820 females per 1000 males in Harayana, while Punjab had 793 females per 1000 males[65]. This clearly shows the continuing drop in the female/male ratio due to the wide use of prenatal genetic diagnosis technology for gender selection, in spite of implemention of a law prohibiting it.

Several IVF specialists offer sex selection as a choice to the couple and do not believe that it amounts to perpetuating male domination and discrimination against the girl child. The new law against sex-selection methods now includes technologies such as PGD, but it remains to be seen whether it is a deterrent.

Recourse to sex selection in India and China, even in defiance of laws, illustrates social settings where son-preference stems from customary practices of discrimination against women and girls. Senior policy-makers in both countries deplore this discrimination, and propose fundamental social reforms to provide gender equality. The paradox or irony, however, is that the cost of prohibition of sex selection, properly viewed as symptomatic of discrimination against women, is borne, for instance in India, disproportionately by women (Dickens *et al.*, in press).

CONCLUSION

Traditions should respect the needs of infertile people. Different religious visions all aim to benefit humanity, satisfying human needs and preserving human dignity, although they may differ in some details which are relevant to basic values in each faith. Policy-makers should be aware of these differences when policy is applied to regulate ART practices. Given the vulnerability of human nature, the task is to work out with the appropriate authorities the means to regulate new practices in sensitive areas such as ART without the intervention of criminal law. The goal of regulation must be to secure maximum freedom of practice and research which are compatible with the interest of patients, their cultural and religious precepts and the common good and values of the society that they inhabit. This pragmatic statement also reflects the belief of all religions discussed. Given the long time required to legislate or amend laws in this rapidly changing field of medicine, it may be better to lay down broad principles and guidelines as a regulatory framework. Practice and research can then be regulated by a code issued by responsible bodies or councils. This code can then be amended from time to time to accommodate any new developments in the field. Meanwhile, it is essential for practicing physicians to be aware of the cultural and religious background of their patients before they offer them advice on different medical practices in ART. It is also essential that a doctor who has conscientious objections to a line of treatment required or requested by the patient should refer the patient elsewhere, where his/her treatment can be performed.

REFERENCES

1. Rabelais F. La Vie de Gargantua et de Pantagruel. 1532.
2. Serour GI. Ethical considerations of assisted reproductive technologies: a Middle Eastern perspective [Opinion]. Middle East Fertil Soc J 2000; 5: 13–18.
3. Genesis 1: 28.
4. Sura Al-Ra'd 13: 38, Holy Qur'an.
5. The book of changes (Yi Jing). In Meng Zi, ed. Four Books and Five Classics. Beijing: China's Bookstore, 1985: 1–55.
6. Ng EHY, Liu A, Chan CHY, et al. Regulating reproductive technology in Hong Kong. J Assist Reprod Genet 2003; 20: 281–6.
7. Steptoe PC, Edwards RG. Birth after the preimplantation of a human embryo. Lancet 1978; 2: 366.
8. Serour GI, Aboulghar MA, Mansour RT. Bioethics in medically assisted conception in the Muslim world. J Assist Reprod Genet 1995; 12: 559–65.
9. Dunstan GR. Diagnosis and treatment of infertility: a religious and ethical discussion. Christian Moral Reasoning. EAGO Congress, Budapest, June 20 1996. EAGO Newslett 1996; 2: 29–31.
10. Shenker JG. Gender selection: cultural and religious perspectives. J Assist Reprod Genet 2002; 19: 400–10.
11. Genesis 19: 11.
12. Genesis 30.
13. Schenker JG. Legal aspects of ART practice in Israel. J Assist Reprod Genet 2003; 20: 250–9.
14. State of Israel Knesset Law. Prohibition of Human Cloning 1999, 2004.
15. Pope Pius XII. Roman Catholic Church, 1956.
16. Cardinal Ratzinger J. Approved by Pope Paul II. Vatican City, 1987.
17. The Talbert 250, 8130. 1 June 1996: 741.
18. Gregorios, Archbishop General for high Coptic studies, cultural and scientific research. Christianity views on IVF and ET in treatment of infertility and test tube babies. In Kamal R, ed. Akhbar El Youm, 1989; 82: 131.
19. The ESHRE Ethics Taskforce, Shenfield F, Pennings G, Devroey P, et al. Taskforce 5: preimplantation genetic diagnosis. Hum Reprod 2003; 18: 649–51.
20. Millot JA. L'art de procréer les sexes à volonté, 4 édn. Vers, 1820.
21. Cohen J. Gender selection: is there a European view? J Assist Reprod Genet 2002; 19: 417–19.

22. Lui P, Rose GA. Social aspects of over 800 couples coming forward for gender selection of their children. Hum Reprod 1995; 10: 968–71.

23. Human Fertilisation and Embryology Authority. Sex Selection: Options for Regulation. London: HFEA, 2003. www.hfea.gov.uk/AboutHFEA/Consultations/

24. Royal Commission on New Technologies. Proceed with care: final report of the Royal Commission. Ottawa, Canada: Minister of Government Services, 1993: 889.

25. McDougall J, De Wit KJ, Ebanks GE. Parental preferences for sex of children in Canada. Sex roles. J Res 1999; 40: 615.

26. Pope John Paul II. Vatican City, 27 November 2001.

27. Gad El Hak AGE, Serour GI, eds. Some Gynecological Problems in the Context of Islam. The International Islamic Center for Population Studies and Research. Cairo: Al-Azhar University, 2000.

28. Serour GI. Attitudes and cultural perspective on infertility and its alleviation in the Middle East Area. In Vayenna E, ed. Current Practices and Controversies in Assisted Reproduction. Report of a WHO Meeting. Geneva: WHO, 2002: 41–9.

29. Sura Al-Bakara 2: 185, Holy Qur'an.

30. Sura Al-Ahzab 32: 4–5, Holy Qur'an.

31. Gad El Hak AGE. In vitro fertilization and test tube baby. Dar El Iftaa, Cairo, Egypt, 1980; 1(115): 3213–28.

32. Proceedings of 7th Meeting of the Islamic Fikh Council in IVF & ET and AIH, Mecca (1984). Kuwait Siasa Daily Newspaper, March 1984.

33. Serour GI. Embryo Research. Ethical implications in the Islamic World. Rabat, Morocco: ISESCO, 2002.

34. Serour GI, ed. Ethical Guidelines for Human Reproduction Research in the Muslim World. The International Islamic Center for Population Studies and Research. Cairo: Al-Azhar University, 1992.

35. Serour GI, ed. Ethical Implications of the Use of ART in the Muslim World. The International Islamic Center for Population Studies and Research. Cairo: Al-Azhar University, 1997.

36. Serour GI, ed. Ethical Implications of the Use of ART in the Muslim World: Update. The International Islamic Center for Population Studies and Research. Cairo: Al-Azhar University, 2000.

37. Islamic Organization of Education, Science and Culture (ISESCO). Ethical Reflection of Advanced Genetic Research. Doha, Qatar: ISESCO, 1993.

38. Serour GI, Dickens B. Assisted reproduction developments in the Islamic World. Int J Gynecol Obstet 2001; 74: 187–93.

39. Tantawi S. Islamic Sharia and Selective Fetal Reduction. Al Ahram Daily Newspaper, Cairo, Egypt, 1991.

40. Sura El Hag 22: 5, Holy Qur'an.

41. Sura El Mómenon 23: 14, Holy Qur'an.

42. Hadith Shareef. Reported by Bokhary and Muslim.

43. Sura Al Nahl 16: 58–9, Holy Qur'an.

44. Sura Al Takwir 81: 8–9, Holy Qur'an.

45. Fathalla MF. The girl child. Int J Gynecol Obstet 2000; 70: 7–12.

46. Serour GI. Transcultural issues in gender selection. In Daya S, Harrison R, Kampers R, eds. Recent Advances in Infertility and Reproductive Technology. International Federation of Fertility Societies (IFFS) 18th World Congress on Fertility and Sterility, Montréal 2004. Amsterdam: Elsevier, 2004.

47.   Serour GI. Family and sex selection. In Healy DL, Kovacs GT, McLachlan R, Rodriguez-Arms O, eds. Reproductive Medicine in the Twenty-first Century. Proceedings of the 17th World Congress on Fertility and Sterility, Melbourne, Australia. London, UK: Parthenon Publishing, 2002: 97–106.

48.   Serour GI. Ethical guidelines for gender selection: are they needed? Presented at the International Conference on Reproductive Disruptions: Childlessness, Adoption, and Other Reproductive Complexities, University of Michigan, Ann Arbor, May 2005.

49.   El Bayoumi AA, Al Ali K. Gene therapy: the state of the art. In Ethical Reflection of Advanced Genetic Research. Rabat, Morocco: ISESCO, 2000.

50.   Ren-Zong Qiu. Socio cultural dimensions of infertility and assisted reproduction in the Far East. In Vayenna E, ed. Current Practices and Controversies in Assisted Reproduction. Report of a WHO Meeting, Geneva: WHO, 2002: 75–80.

51.   Chen HW, Tao J. Moral exploration of whether surrogate motherhood should be comprehensively prohibited in Hong Kong. In Tao J, Ren-Zong Qiu, eds. Value and Society. Beijing: Chinese Social Sciences Press, 1997: 137–55.

52.   Li D. Preference for sons: past and present. China Population Today 1997; 14: 15–16.

53.   Liu NCA. Family law for the Hong Kong SAR. Hong Kong: Hong Kong University Press, 1999.

54.   Wang Y. The impact of boy preference on fertility in China. Chin J Popul Sci 1996; 8: 69–75.

55.   Chan CLW, Yip PSF, Ng EHY, et al. Gender selection in China, its meanings and implications. J Assist Reprod Genet 2002; 19: 426–30.

56.   Cook RJ, Dickens BM, Fathalla MF. Reproductive Health and Human Rights: Integrating Medicine, Ethics and Law. Oxford: Oxford University Press, 2003: 196–202.

57.   Ren-Zong Qiu. Institute of Philosophy, Chinese Academy of Social Science. Action recommendations on correcting the birth sex ratio imbalance. Beijing: Chinese Academy of Social Sciences, 2004.

58.   Widge A. Social cultural attitudes towards infertility and assisted reproduction in India. In Vayenna E, ed. Current Practices and Controversies in Assisted Reproduction. Report of a WHO Meeting. Geneva: WHO, 2002: 60–74.

59.   Allahabadia GN, Kaur K. Accreditation, supervision, and regulation of ART clinics in India – a distant dream? J Assist Reprod Genetics 2003; 20: 276–80.

60.   Jindal UN, Gupta AN. Social problems of infertility in women in India. Int J Fertil 1989; 30: 30–3.

61.   Gupta J. New Reproductive Technologies, Women's Health and Autonomy: Freedom or Dependence? New Delhi: Sage Publications, 2000.

62.   Bhargava PM. Ethical issues in modern biological technologies. Reprod Biomed Online 2003; 7: 276–85.

63.   Kumar K. Amniocentesis and gender discrimination in India. In Kegley, KAJ, ed. Genetic Knowledge: Human Values and Responsibility. Kentucky: Lexington, 1998: 147–66.

64.   Mudur G. Indian medical authorities act on antenatal sex selection. Br Med J 1999; 319: 401.

65.   Registrar General of India. Provisional Population Totals, Census of India 2001, New Delhi, Office of the Registrar General of India. 2001, www.censusindia.net/results-main.

Index